# Self-Care for Life in the City

## How to nourish your mind, body and soul in a fast-paced world

*by*
*Francesca Blechner*

First Printed in United Kingdom 2020

Published by Conscious Dreams Publishing
www.consciousdreamspublishing.com

Cover Illustration by Jae Thompson

Cover Design by Alaka Oladimeji Basit

Edited by Rhoda Molife
.www.molahmedia.com

Typeset by Nadia Vitushynska

Foreword by Paul Chek, Founder of The C.H.E.K. Institute

Author Photograph by Oba Otite of Obti-cat-ion

ISBN: 978-1-912551-97-2

## Dedication

This book is dedicated to all the teachers, coaches and mentors I've had in my life — your teachings have inspired me to write this book. To all my clients, past and present, I have learnt so much from you and am grateful and humbled to be a part of your life's journey.

# Testimonials

*I am in awe of Fran's dedication and commitment to her craft. She is a true force in the world of holistic wellbeing and an advocate of living a long life full of energy and balance. Fran's driven by the need to restore balance and inner wellbeing to mind, body and soul. A complete understanding of humans on all levels and how the mind, body and soul are connected is essential to healing ourselves completely. Fran has this knowledge and wisdom in spades. She is a much-needed fresh voice in a world full of stress, pressure and disconnection. I've no doubt this book will be a huge success.*

**Jody Shield, Performance and Business Coach for Entrepreneurs, TEDx Speaker, Author and Podcaster**

*'I've worked with Fran for a number of years and after every session I feel as if my mind and body have been recalibrated for the day ahead. She has a very intuitive and calming approach that is perfectly suited to a stressed-out ad executive with small children and minimal time. My hour with Fran has kept my nervous system in check in an often hectic week.'*

**Sonny Adorjan, Creative Director**

*'Francesca has that rare balance of supreme and forthright confidence coupled with real empathy. I found myself really opening up, being truly honest with myself and embracing a significant amount of change — all of which have had measurable and sustainable improvements on my health and well-being.'*

**James Kowszun, COO Bibendum**

*'I was going through an overwhelmingly challenging period in my life when I decided to work with Francesca, and it made an incredible difference. Francesca is very skilful, patient, caring and attentive to detail and has a thorough understanding of the mind-body connection. She helped to restore balance where harmony had been disturbed.'*

**Enrida Kelly, Founder, NATPATH Clinic and Co-Author of *Healing Cancer***

'I was feeling incredibly frustrated, physically exhausted and emotionally drained. Working with Fran, I gained a huge amount of clarity and direction for my business venture. I realised just how important it was to have the foundations of health, stress management, sleep, nutrition, movement and rest firmly in place before even considering making any serious lifestyle changes.'

**Leigh Jones, Wellbeing Coach**

'Francesca is one of the most intuitive facilitators I know. She's an absolute joy to work with and has an in-depth knowledge and experience of the body and the nervous system.'

**Rebecca Dennis, Founder of Breathing Tree and Author of *And Breathe***

'This lady literally transformed my life. Her knowledge is outstanding, and she is clearly passionate about helping people. I've deepened my spirituality and connection to self. I have known and worked with Fran for years and she continually impresses me with her dedication to her work.'

**Angela Graham, CHEK Holistic Lifestyle Coach & Movement Specialist**

'I was really struggling to balance full-time work and being a mum. The stress was causing me debilitating back and neck pain. Working with Fran, I have learnt tools and techniques to improve my breathing, refocus my energies and care for my mind and body together. I now feel in a better place for anything that life throws at me!'

**Jane D, Senior Project Support**

'This book is a comprehensive personal growth experience, full of scientific explanation and answers to most questions with examples and practical exercises. Her work is truly transformational and will inspire others to make life changing decisions. Her conviction that mind, body and spirit must walk along together makes us have a complete experience of what life can become: a journey of pleasant discoveries about ourselves, full of joy, awareness, acceptance and peace, even if you live in a big city. This is a must-read!'

**Hanna Meirelles, Co-Author #1 Amazon bestseller *Ignite your Life for Conscious Leaders*; Global Trainer and Development Facilitator and Founder of Life Level 10**

# Foreword

*by Paul Chek, Founder of The C.H.E.K institute*

We are living in a time of a deeper exploration of the human mind and its great powers of diversity. School starts early and our heads are filled with many ideas we must memorise to pass tests. Often though, these ideas don't turn out to be of any practical assistance to living in a modern world, or realizing what actually creates and supports life. We can make computers, but have forgotten how to eat, move, breathe, and rest effectively.

As humans, we use our complex mental abilities to explore various domains of knowledge; while we invent some things that are helpful to and harmonious with our natural surroundings, we invent many more that are dangerous to our health and to nature, the latter being essential to support our existence. Imagine being smart enough to genetically engineer food crops that produce their own pesticides and overlook the fact that any creature or human eating them will be immediately poisoned and damaged.

The stories we were once told — now called myths — by our elders were there to help us understand the mysteries of life, relate to each other, grasp the inevitable stages of life from birth to death and realize ourselves as part of a grand whole — The Cosmos. Where we once gathered in groups to share our experiences of the mystical and create more love and wholeness together, we now have ethnocentric belief systems designed to profit a few and control the masses by inducing fear. The degradation of our connection to nature and each other resulting from an academic, scientific dissection of our myths reducing them to ridiculous stories, or worse yet, lies, has led to the modern myth of consumerism; today, people fruitlessly seek happiness by purchasing things endlessly, hoping for connection, safety, and security...something to fill the void that was once filled by our magical relationship with nature.

Technology has advanced rapidly, and with it, the speed of information transfer and the abundance of information we each deal with. The result is that today, most people are very confused about how to eat for their individual needs, what exercises are best for them, why sticking to natural cycles are essential for our regeneration. Above all they prostitute themselves to jobs in which they make *money, not love.*

In this beautiful book, **Self-Care for Life In The City**, Francesca Blechner shares a synthesis of timeless truths we can all use to find and create our dreams, live well, and be conscious of what is ultimately important and sustainable.

I have personally engaged these principles my whole life, being fortunate enough to have been raised by a mother that practices yoga, and a father that is a farmer; my parents taught us what is essential, why it is essential, and grounded us in the very types of principles Francesca shares with you here.

With just a little effort each day to apply the holistic teachings in this book, you will find yourself having more energy, mental clarity, creativity and compassion for all living beings; you will surely come to realize that to be healthy, we must all make purchases that fund sustainable farming and manufacturing processes.

As you detoxify yourself, you will become aware (often for the first time) that what you once thought was a cost-effective way of eating or living was ultimately not saving you at all. The toxins you are clearing for your own health and well-being are also rampant in nature due to the short-sightedness of the corporations producing 'cheap foods and produce'. Your wireless devices may make it easier to communicate and be entertained, but that all changes when electromagnetic pollution disrupts normal brain function, overheats and inflames your body, leading to a potentially endless stream of doctor visits and prescription drugs to treat the symptoms of *'an easier life'*.

The beauty of this book is that it is simple and direct; in just a few hours, you can rewrite the blueprint for your self-management and begin living a life of awareness, vitality allowing you to become a healing force in the world.

I hope you enjoy **Self-Care for Life In The City** as much as I have.

Love and chi,
Paul Chek
Holistic Health Practitioner
Founder, C.H.E.K Institute
Founder, PPS Success Mastery Program

# Contents

# Introduction

We are living in a time where stress is at an all-time high in the city due to lifestyle and environmental factors. Poor quality food, contaminated water, environmental stress, demanding work hours, perfectionism and a lack of time for self, have taken over so many people's lives. Most people that I've worked with who are living in the city are either overwhelmed, suffering from exhaustion, fatigued or on the road to burnout.

We've become a nation that runs to the doctor for every minor ailment, ache and pain. Most of us have forgotten how to tune into the innate wisdom of our bodies, how to self-regulate our nervous systems and apply simple ways to take care of ourselves and our minds. Statistics show that one in two people will get cancer[1]; this is not good enough, nor should it be acceptable. Only a small percentage of cancers, and indeed all diseases are genetically inherited. Through the study of epigenetics, we know that environmental and lifestyle factors can determine whether a gene is expressed or not and what possible impact that can have on the development of a disease. So, that means our lifestyle has an impact on our health. If we can learn how to take care of ourselves, we not only have a positive impact on our health but also that of our children and future generations to come.

I started out in the health and fitness industry as a personal trainer in 2001, working all hours of the day and eventually bringing myself to the edge of burnout many times. There was no doubt that I loved what I did but I was running on adrenaline and exhausting myself. In my early 30s, I came to a crossroads, feeling really stuck, overwhelmed, anxious and fearful of moving forward. Fitness focused mainly on one aspect of health — the physical — with little regard to mental, emotional and spiritual health. With a thirst for knowledge and love of studying, I went on to train in many holistic modalities, including holistic lifestyle coaching with the CHEK Institute, Transformational Breath®, teaching yoga, Wildfitness coaching, abdominal massage, neuromuscular

---

1   1 in 2 people in the UK will get cancer (2015) — www.cancerresearchuk.org/about-us/cancer-news/press-release/2015-02-04-1-in-2-people-in-the-uk-will-get-cancer

activation and various bodywork techniques that demonstrated how emotional states manifest in the body. During this time, I was forced to re-evaluate my life and the pace at which I was living. Following one of my trainings, I felt 'drunk for a week' after my nervous system went into a complete reboot, forcing me to rest!

In my 20 years of working in well-being, I have noticed a monumental increase in the number of people with burnout, adrenal fatigue, auto-immune disease, anxiety and trauma. As the pace of life and technology has increased immensely during this time, we are trying to live at a speed that human physiology has simply not adapted to. It's time to take back our power and ownership for our health and happiness. The body is the only place we're guaranteed to live in our whole lives. We have to look after it, nourish it and simply love it. The more we begin to connect back with our mind, body and soul using some of the self-care practices in this book, the stronger our relationship with self will be. It then becomes easier to make loving, healthy choices that nourish us in our entirety.

Attempting to make big changes to health and well-being overnight often feels overwhelming, setting oneself up for self-sabotaging behaviours. I like to use the analogy of a bank, a health bank; this means making deposits that are adding value to your health and well-being and letting them accumulate over time just like you would your bank account. Your withdrawals are those things that are taking away from your health, let's say a big blow-out of alcohol. However, instead of feeling guilty and berating yourself the next day, look at where you can maximise your deposits. You can drink lots of high-quality water, have a green juice with parsley and lemon to help cleanse the liver, or go to bed on time the following night. You will find my health bank deposit tips at the end of each section.

You see, the aim is not to live a life of perfection where you berate yourself if you 'slip up'. The idea is to adopt lifestyle behaviours that increase your resilience so much in mind, body and soul that your stress tolerance is set much higher and you move from surviving to thriving in the city.

The time is now. Self-care is not an option any more, nor is it an indulgence; it is a necessity for the human species to survive and thrive. I have seen and witnessed through my career as a holistic practitioner too many people simply burnout. The most common factors for this are stress, chemical stress, lifestyle and unresolved emotional blockages, and people of all ages are now vulnerable.

It's my passion to help others thrive physically, mentally, emotionally and spiritually, and to live in alignment with the life they desire. Through the practices I share with you in this book, I feel the happiest and most fulfilled I've ever been. I'm living in alignment with my vision, values and purpose. I'm living at a pace where I feel grounded, resilient and can thrive rather than survive.

My wish is for you to have the same.

With love and gratitude,

Francesca

# PART 1

# The Mind

## The Modern-Day Stress Epidemic

Government national statistics from the Health and Safety Executive (HSE) reported 12.8 million working days were lost due to work-related stress, depression or anxiety in 2018 / 19 across the UK[2], with Londoners having the highest levels of anxiety[3].

Most people I come across today are struggling to keep up with themselves. They are 'hanging in there' and just about keeping their heads above water. They are putting so much energy out and yet are unable to replenish and cultivate their life force to the same degree. They are constantly stimulated and 'switched on', which if unchecked leads to burnout. Think about your phone battery; if it's always on and being used, the battery runs out and eventually it has to be recharged. Humans are the same; we need to recharge our batteries.

The *autonomic nervous system* controls our bodies without us even being aware. It is split into two pathways. One is the *sympathetic nervous system* which controls the body's response to dangerous or stressful situations with the help of hormones like cortisol, adrenaline and noradrenaline; it gives us our 'get up and go.' Then there is the *parasympathetic nervous system* which controls our organs and processes like digestion, heart rate, the immune response, rest, repair and breathing; it acts in opposition to the sympathetic nervous system, keeping our functions under control.

We need stress — it gives us our get up and go to get stuff done. However, most people I come across in the city are wired and tired! Their sympathetic nervous system is constantly stimulated, and they are operating on a constant level of fight / flight / freeze (FFF). To paint a picture, since the dawn of time, the FFF response was useful in the event of acute danger such as being faced with a tiger, fighting a tribe or any other life-and-death situation. In these acute moments, the digestive

---

2   Health and Safety Executive: Work-related stress, anxiety or depression statistics in Great Britain (2019) — www.hse.gov.uk/statistics/causdis/stress.pdf
3   London Mental Health (2014) — www.london.gov.uk/sites/default/files/gla_migrate_files_destination/Mental%20health%20report.pdf

and reproductive systems shut down, as in that moment, they are not essential for survival. Glucose (sugar) is dumped into the muscles for energy should one have to run for their life...or fight the tiger. Blood pressure and heart rate increase, pupils dilate and the stress hormones cortisol and adrenaline are pumped into the body. This is called the stress response and is known to suppress the immune system. Once the threat disappears, all recovers in 24 – 48 hours.

Our physiology is hard-wired since the days of our primal ancestors and does not know the difference between the stress of facing a tiger and the accumulated stresses of daily life. The stress response is thus the same. The pressure to achieve, strive to do and be more, lack of sleep, work, relationship and financial issues, a poor diet, busy commutes, endless notifications, lack of sunshine and digital bombardment are more prevalent than ever. These factors and stresses are cumulative and with all these triggers going on throughout each day, the stress response is constantly stimulated. If it is not balanced out with enough quiet time and rest, it can lead to chronic inflammation and a suppressed immune system for one. The consequences are chronic ill health and thus you can see the importance of lifestyle changes to reduce stress.

There are two forms of stress: *situational* or *emotional* and *physiological*.

*Situational stress* triggers are:
- Family issues
- Relationships
- Financial worries
- Moving home
- Death of a loved one

The resultant feelings of grief, anxiety, frustration, sadness, loneliness and depression all trigger a stress response.

There are six forms of *physiological stress*, all of which are prevalent in the city. They impact on the physiology — the function of the body:

- **Nutritional** — processed and chemically sprayed foods and contaminated water.

- **Chemical** — toxic chemicals sprayed on food, chemicals from household cleaning products and cosmetics.

- **Environmental** — heavy metals from air and water pollution.

   The build-up of these stresses can overwhelm the liver, the organ that breaks down waste. The burden becomes too much, the adrenal glands come under pressure and the stress response is triggered. Those suffering from auto-immune disease, chronic fatigue, fibromyalgia and burnout are often very sensitive to chemicals and environmental stressors.

- **Postural** — spending long hours sitting at a desk with minimum movement and sub-optimal breathing patterns puts stress and pressure on the organs and joints.

- **Mental** — taking on high workloads, focusing on lack and what you don't want and increased anxiety.

- **Electromagnetic** — radiation from Wi-Fi, mobile phones, power lines and phone masts. Most people working in an office are bombarded by electromagnetic fields.

Ultimately, whatever the stressor the effect is the same on the autonomic nervous system. This book addresses all these factors by addressing the six foundational pillars of health: breathing, thoughts, water, nutrition, rest and movement. It gives simple strategies and easy-to-implement actions bringing conscious awareness to the thoughts we think and the lifestyle choices we make. The ultimate aim is to serve towards a better you, improved health and that of the planet.

# Values and Redefining Success

*'We sacrifice our health in order to make wealth, then we sacrifice our wealth in order to get back our health.'* — Dalai Lama

Traditionally, being successful meant having a good job with a fancy title, money, a big house, nice car and more. This is the standard we are set and we go to school, work hard, get good grades and go to university to achieve this standard. However, more often than not, what happens is that you come out with lots of debt, broken promises of a full-time career in your field and you usually end up working for someone else's dream. I recently met a very 'successful' corporate lawyer on paper who often worked long into the night, at times sleeping in the office only to be back at his desk at 8am. When I asked how he relaxed, his answer was 'I fall asleep on the sofa in front of the TV.' Is a job that pays well with a fancy title but one that demands long hours leaving little time for yourself really worth the expense of your health, happiness, relationships and social time?

> Begin thinking of your *time* and *energy* as your most valuable commodities; you can never get back your time. Once it's gone, it's gone. Choose how you spend your time wisely.

While studying my holistic lifestyle coaching course with CHEK Europe[4], one activity we had to do was identify our top three priorities and our core values. I surprised myself because I didn't have a clear response to this. I vaguely knew what they were and so I was getting vague results in my life and attracting vague relationships. Not quite knowing what direction I was headed, I felt permanently overwhelmed, confused and ungrounded. With the ability to quieten my mind and listen to my intuition, I was able to list my top three priorities which I live by today. Here they are:

1. *My health* — my health is my wealth. I firmly believe this; having vibrant health changes the way I move, feel and operate in the world.

---

4  The CHEK Institute — www.chekinstitute.com

2. *Living from a place of passion and purpose* — these fuel the fire inside me and make me feel truly alive.

3. *Love and relationships* — I spend time with those that I have nurturing meaningful, loving relationships with, including myself.

When I ask my clients what the core values of their business or workplace are, they can quickly tell me, but when asking for themselves, they too struggle to come up with an answer. To clarify, priorities are external principles guided by your internal values — these include family, business, finances etc. Core values are personalised and guide the way you live your life — your lifestyle choices, the way you work and your overall life principles and perceptions. All values must be acted upon or you are not living in alignment with them.

List your top three priorities below and the reason why they are:

1. Connection — quality over quantity, honest, stimulating, on same wavelength

2. Wellness — emotional strength, clarity, calm, joy, inspiration, balance, time, no rushing

3. Creating — plas, colour, reflection, in all forms, expression process.

Look at your top three priorities. Is there something there for you? Often, people will give their energy and power to everything else but themselves — job, partner, children, for example, with nothing left for themselves. Is this you? If so, you will soon become depleted so go back and re-evaluate your priorities. Fill your cup up first and then give others from the overflow.

20

Now, write out at least three core values for each one. For example:

1. **My health**
   - I meditate daily to keep me centred
   - I eat good, high-quality, organic foods, applying the 80:20 rule
   - I go to bed by 10.30pm at least four times a week to feel really energised and rested
2. **Living from a place of passion and purpose**
   - I do work that lights my heart and soul
   - I invest in my personal and professional development to continually grow and be inspired
   - I take time out to travel and experience new things that excite me
3. **Love and relationships (including your relationship with you)**
   - I meet up with a friend once a week
   - I have an evening to myself at home at least once a week to self-nurture
   - My partner and I share similar values.

When you become clear about your priorities and values, you'll also become more aware of your behaviours and whether they match or deflect those values. You then align with the real *you*. Without values you're like a seaman with a malfunctioning compass trying to navigate the waters in unpredictable weather. Once you become clear on what your values are, your internal compass aligns giving you direction and the ability to navigate your journey regardless of the external circumstances. When you are clear on your priorities and values you can reach your desired results much more quickly.

As you write down your values, think about where you need to implement and want to experience more of these values in your life. How are you demonstrating these values? If for example your priority is vibrant health but you are eating greasy takeaways every other night, then this is sending confusing and conflicting messages to your subconscious. Instead, what you can do to feel vibrantly healthy is prioritise having a few key healthy ingredients at the beginning of the week readily available in the fridge. That way you can always put a healthy meal together quickly and not be tempted by fast food.

Clarifying your values allows you to redefine success for *yourself*, not what society, your parents, peers or your colleagues think it is for you. You and you alone are in control of your destiny and your compass — your values — will take you there. Take back your power, get back in the driving seat and enjoy the game of life. It is important to regularly check in on your values too. Remember they may change over time as you continually evolve. As you cement them into daily living however, you gain clarity on the things you want to attract. I thoroughly recommend sitting down and writing your core values for every area of your life: lifestyle, health, relationships, work, family, home, finances and self-care.

### My definition of success is:

*'I choose to live my life with joy, passion and purpose. I have vibrant, radiant health and energy so that I can be the container to facilitate transformation, make a difference and impact as many people's lives as I can. I am happy and fulfilled with the work I bring to the world. I have the energy and time to do the things I love and spend time with those I love.'*

Write out your definition of success for you. It can be as short or as long as you like. Put it somewhere that you can easily see it so that it's a daily reminder. Mine is on my wall next to my bed.

### My definition of success:

*I live as an artist, my art is my
priority. I am boundaried, I nurture
the highest quality connections. I
give myself all the time &
support I need to be the best
version of me*

### Health Bank Deposit

✓ Identify your top three priorities

✓ Write at least three to five core values for each priority

✓ Write out your own definition of success for yourself and put it somewhere where you can see it daily.

## The Power of Your Thoughts

We are multi-dimensional beings made up of mind, body and spirit. The mind is divided into the *conscious, subconscious* and *unconscious.* Freud, the father of psychoanalysis, refers to the mind as being like an iceberg, with the conscious mind being the tip of the iceberg that emerges just above the water (*Freud, 2001*). The conscious mind consists of everything inside your awareness; it is the mental processing that allows us to think, talk and rationalise. The subconscious mind, which sits just below the surface of the water, consists of fears, desires, emotions and memories that we are not fully aware of but can pull into the conscious mind when required. Let's say someone asks you what you had for dinner last night. While you may not be walking around actively thinking about what you ate last night, you can quickly get the information if required. Self-limiting beliefs also live in the subconscious. Freud refers to the subconscious mind as the gatekeeper between the conscious and unconscious.

The unconscious mind is the bulk of the iceberg underneath the surface of the water; it's the feelings, desires, memories and emotions that the unconscious mind wants to keep hidden and repressed from awareness. Often, deep-rooted trauma is stored and 'forgotten' here. It is said that the unconscious mind governs more of our emotions and actions than we realise but is much more challenging to access.

Ninety-five percent of brain activity is beyond our conscious awareness, thus most people are running their lives from the programming in their subconscious mind (*Zaltman, 2003*). It's like the operating system of a computer running its program. Your life reflects the programs in your mind, which are the beliefs developed over time under the influence of education, family, religion, peers, society and the media.

*'Thoughts are things.'* — Napoleon Hill

Thoughts are powerful. Thoughts create your reality. Have you ever taken the time to monitor your thoughts and the relentless self-chatter running through your mind? It's important to be aware of your thoughts and consider whether they are serving you, moving you forwards or keeping you stuck and in fear?

*'Your worst enemy cannot harm you as much as your unguarded thoughts.*
*Happiness does not depend on what you have or who you are.*
*It solely relies on what you think.' —* Buddha

Deepak Chopra, an advocate of alternative medicine, says that we have an estimated 60,000 to 80,000 thoughts a day, most of which are disempowering and self-sabotaging.[5] Imagine having a friend who was constantly following you around berating you, telling you 'you're not good enough', 'you're too fat', 'you're not attractive enough', 'you look stupid', 'you're not lovable', 'you're useless'. Chances are you would soon get rid of that so-called friend. Yet, how many of us have this constant negative self-talk running through our minds without even being aware of it and accepting that it's okay to talk to yourself like that?

There is a French advert by Dove called the inner critic which demonstrates this beautifully[6]. A group of women were asked to write down every time they had a bad thought about themselves in a notebook. They were then invited back to a cafe for coffee. In the cafe was an actress who appeared to be talking to a friend, repeating the women's recorded bad thoughts. Strangers in the cafe interrupted the conversation to tell the actress that she was being very harsh. The women, who recognised their thoughts being spoken aloud, were horrified when they realised the power behind their thoughts and how damaging they were. If those words were not acceptable to say to someone else, why are they acceptable to say it to themselves?! I recommend you watch it.

*'You are a living magnet and you inevitably attract into your life the*
*people, circumstances, ideas and resources in harmony with your*
*dominant thoughts.' —* Brian Tracy

Pay attention to your thoughts and ensure you are talking and thinking about what you want, rather than what you don't want. The same goes for what you feed your mind with, especially those subliminal messages that come from what you watch, listen to or read. If the first thing you do when you wake up is switch on the news and

5  Why meditate? (2013) — www.chopra.com/articles/why-meditate-0
6  Dove France, Inner Critic Commercial — https://www.youtube.com/watch?v=MOLike-Hkpg

hear the doom and gloom of the world, then that's likely to evoke fear-based emotions and feelings that carry over into your day. Likewise, when taking public transport or the tube to work, which can be stressful enough in rush-hour, avoid reading the newspaper; rarely do you see headlines in conventional newspapers that are happy and joyful. Often, I've had clients tell me that they arrive at work in an anxious state, having jumped out of bed late, eaten breakfast out the door, and squashed into a packed tube with no breathing space all topped off with the misery of the happenings in the world. How you start your day is key to how the rest of your day flows. Many great leaders, speakers and entrepreneurs talk of morning rituals: owning your morning means owning the day. We'll explore this more in Part Three — Creating a Morning Ritual.

*'We become what we think about most of the time.'* — Earl Nightingale

Dr David Hamilton, author of *The Five Side-Effects of Kindness*, researched stress and kindness (*Hamilton, 2017*). His findings showed that kindness has the opposite effect to stress. A kind thought, act or gesture that puts a smile on your face literally soothes the body.

| STRESS | KINDNESS |
|---|---|
| Creates stress hormones (like cortisol and adrenaline) | Creates 'molecules of kindness' (oxytocin and nitric oxide) |
| Creates tension in the nervous system | Relaxes the nervous system (by increasing vagal tone) |
| Increases blood pressure | Reduces blood pressure |
| Generates free radicals (oxidative stress) and inflammation | Reduces free radicals (oxidative stress) and inflammation |
| Linked with cardiovascular disease | Kindness is cardioprotective |
| Weakens the immune system | Boosts the immune system |
| Associated with unhappiness | Boosts happiness |
| Linked with depression | Protects against depression |
| Accelerates ageing | Slows ageing |

\* From research cited in David A Hamilton, PhD, *The Five Side Effects of Kindness*

We will explore thoughts, feelings, manifestations and the law of attraction further in Part Three.

### Retraining the Subconscious Mind

Start by paying attention to your thoughts and bringing awareness to the recurring thoughts running through your mind daily. Can you identify the top three thoughts that are not serving you?

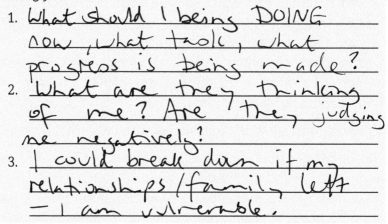

1. What should I being DOING now, what task, what progress is being made?
2. What are they thinking of me? Are they judging me negatively?
3. I could break down if my relationships/family left — I am vulnerable.

When we are constantly thinking we cannot be in the present moment.

*'Your past is growing every day as you go on accumulating thoughts, memories and experiences. Every day you have a bigger and bigger mind (the computer operating system) and less and less consciousness.'* —
Osho, Indian Spiritual Master

Osho says that when we live moment to moment, dying to the past and to expectations of the future, we become more present, opening a new space within and expanding consciousness.

### Health Bank Deposits

✓ Become aware of your daily thoughts
✓ Identify the top three thoughts that are not serving you. In the next section, we will replace these with affirmations.
✓ Watch the Dove Inner Critic commercial

# The Power of 'I Am'

*'I AM are the two most powerful words,*
*for what you put after them shapes your reality.' —*
Bevan Lee, Australian TV Script Writer and Executive

Internationally renowned author and speaker the late Dr Wayne Dyer speaks much of the power of *I am* (*Dyer, 2012*). When you speak in the *I am*, you are speaking of your true being; no one else can say *I am* for you. What follows *I am* can determine your reality, limit or free you. You are speaking in the present tense and declaring loud and clear to the universe, right now, what you are.

As discussed earlier, you have 60,0000 to 80,000 thoughts a day, most of which are not serving you. The *I am* is working throughout the day. If you are saying to yourself 'I am so old', 'I am overweight', 'I am ugly' or, 'I am useless', 'I am so clumsy', 'I am rubbish', you are inviting more into your life that makes you feel old, overweight, unattractive, useless, etc; life will give you proof of what you are affirming to be true. Accept where you are right now on your journey with love, compassion and kindness. When you start to bring conscious awareness to your thoughts, you can choose to empower yourself.

### I Am Affirmations

The word 'affirmation' comes from the Latin *affirmare* — to make steady and strengthen.

The brain responds to positive, present-tense statements. It does not know the difference between what is real and false and as you repeat the *I am* positive affirmations you are declaring out loud to the universe that this is truth. The brain is a creature of habit and the more you repeat the affirmations and feel into it, the more it will strengthen the neural connections in the brain of your newly stated truth. This is known as neuroplasticity. You have to train the brain, just like you would a muscle.

I created my own *I am* affirmations that resonated with me about a year ago, and they have had a powerful impact on my life. They've crowded out the subconscious negative thoughts of *I am not* that were running the program! If a negative self-belief does creep in, I can quickly interrupt it, switching to an empowering *I am* affirmation. This comes with time and with nurturing a conscious awareness of your thoughts. It's important to choose the affirmations that resonate with you and evoke a good feeling. Let's say you state an affirmation and your ego says, 'What a load of rubbish,' or 'Who do you think you are?'; instead choose something that evokes a feeling you can connect with. Soon, your self-limiting beliefs will be crowded out.

Here are some examples:
- I am so blessed; blessings always come my way
- I am vibrant, radiant and in good health
- I am powerful
- I am worthy of the best that love, and life have to offer
- I am deserving of success
- I am abundant in health, well-being, friendships and finances
- I am courageous and I stand up for myself
- I am prosperous
- I am open to new opportunities
- I am beautiful
- I am in love with life
- I am powerful beyond measure

Choose three from the above or create your own, write them on a Post-it® note and stick them somewhere you will see them easily and daily. I post some on my fridge and in my bedroom. Remember it must evoke a feeling aligned with what you are stating and ensure you connect with the affirmation; that's where the power is!

Write your three affirmations here:

1. I PAUSE to check in with my needs.

2. I judge me as JUST FINE. I stand still in my POWER. I'm just here DOING ME. I DO ME.

3. I am STRONG, and always choose life.

Now go back and revisit the top three thoughts that are not serving you on page 26 and write the opposite and affirming thought. Remember it must resonate with you and you have to feel it. For example, if the thought 'I am not well' is always running the show, going directly to 'I am radiating vibrant health' may not resonate with you just yet. Instead, I invite you to create an affirmation that bridges the gap such as, 'Every day I am getting better and better' or 'My health is improving every day'.

### Health Bank Deposits

✓ Create three *I am* affirmations for yourself, write them on a Post-it note and place them where you can easily see them every day

✓ Look back at the top three thoughts that are not serving you on page 26 and write the affirmation that negates them.

## The Power of the Breath

The average person takes 17,000 – 23,000 breaths per day.[7] If we don't breathe, we die. So it makes sense to pay attention to the breath, to do breathing exercises and exercise the diaphragm. Our breath pattern is unique and how we breathe is a reflection of how we live life. Breathing affects every single physiological system in the body and can instantly change your emotional state.

### Diaphragmatic Breathing

*'The diaphragm is the body's chief biological pump. If the diaphragm stops working properly, gland and organ function diminish!'* — Paul Chek, Founder of The CHEK Institute

The diaphragm is a dome-shaped sheet of muscle that sits underneath the ribcage. Diaphragmatic breathing can also be known as deep, belly or abdominal breathing. When you inhale, the diaphragm contracts and flattens, pushing the organs downwards and creating a vacuum for air to rush into the lungs. When you exhale, the diaphragm relaxes, and the air is pushed out of the lungs. When breathing properly using your diaphragm, with each inhalation the diaphragm gives the organs an internal massage as it moves downwards. This is deeply nourishing as it increases blood flow to the organs especially the digestive system, all whilst opening up the whole respiratory system. Most people are not using anywhere near the full potential of their lung capacity because we limit ourselves to shallow or chest breathing.

Diaphragmatic breathing activates the parasympathetic nervous system, signalling to the mind and body that it is safe. This lowers the stress response, heart rate, and has even been shown to lower and stabilise high blood pressure.[8] It can also help decrease the levels of cortisol that is released into the body. On the other hand, shallow breathing limits the diaphragm's range of motion and creates tightness

---

7  Harvard Health Publishing Breathing Lessons (2019) — www.health.harvard.edu/mind-and-mood/breathing-lessons

8  Harvard Health Publishing, Harvard Medical School (2015) — 'Relaxation techniques: Breath control helps quell errant stress response' www.health.harvard.edu/mind-and-mood/relaxation-techniques-breath-control-helps-quell-errant-stress-response

in the diaphragm and around the thoracic spine, often leading to lower back pain. When I work with my clients to correct structural issues in their posture, I always release the diaphragm and this often sorts out a lot of back, shoulder and hip issues.

### Grounding Breath Exercise

Find a quiet space and lie on your back with your knees bent. Place one hand on your lower belly and one hand on your chest. Observe what happens when you inhale. Are you breathing into your chest or your abdomen? Is it shallow or is it deep? Is it laboured, or does it feel easy? Observe without judgement and don't try to change it. Observe your breath pattern as it is right now.

Now take a deep breath into the belly and exhale out through the mouth, feeling your body drop heavier into the ground, stretching the jaw open a few times to release any tension. The jaw is another area that stores a lot of tension, tightness and suppressed emotions, particularly anger and frustration. Take a breath into the lower belly through the nose, feel your belly inflate and expand and then exhale out through the nose, feeling the belly relax and drop. Keep the exhalation relaxed and effortless — no blowing out or clenching of the abdominal muscles. The belly moves first and then the chest. I like to imagine the sound of the breath as that of the tide coming in on the inhalation and going out on the exhalation. Try it — it's very soothing. Repeat for ten breaths, closing your eyes and tuning in to the feedback your mind, body and soul are giving you. I often remind my clients to check in throughout the day to see where their breath is. You can do this standing up too — just feel your feet on the ground, allowing your weight to drop down into the hips and pelvis and taking a deep breath into the belly, expanding the lower abdomen. This is a great way to ground your energy and feel more centred.

> *'Taking deep breaths can voluntarily regulate your autonomic nervous system'.* — Jewell

One of my clients, Chris, works hard in finance in the city and often experienced high anxiety and panic attacks. Learning how to self-regulate his autonomic nervous system through breathing was a game-changer for him. Lying down and deep-belly breathing in a dark room became one of his favourite things to do. It allowed him to become aware when his feelings and emotions were triggered and reduce feelings of anxiety through breathing. Taking time to deep-belly breathe daily has increased his resilience and he now has far fewer panic attacks.

As previously mentioned, everyone has a unique breath pattern and your breath pattern mirrors your emotional state. When pain or trauma is experienced, whether physical or emotional, the breath is held. Psychiatrist and author of *The Body Keeps the Score* Bessel Van der Kolk also goes on to say that trauma and it's resulting stress physiologically affects the body and brain and memories get trapped in the body (*Van der Kolk, 2015*).

The natural pattern is to breathe in and out of the belly; when you look at animals, babies and toddlers, you will see their belly moving up and down with each inhale and exhale. However, as we go through our life experiences and are programmed by society, authority figures and peers, it may not feel safe to express our emotions and feelings. How many times have you heard the phrase 'man up', 'don't be a pussy', 'big boys don't cry,' etc. The result? A society of men that are emotionally shut down and checked out, unable to express themselves for fear of being judged as not being a man. They can then turn to alcohol, drugs, porn, sex or crime to numb out and avoid feeling.

Slowly, this is beginning to change though. With a new wave of conscious awakening and well-being, more and more men are seeking yoga, meditation, breath work and self-care. I have been to and facilitated at breath circles where men, young and old, have had the space to release their emotions, cry and integrate these emotions through the power of the breath. I have come across male peers of mine in my training and been shocked at how many of them have been suicidal or even tried to take their own lives. It touches my heart to witness the power of vulnerability, to be able to break through limitations that have been holding them back — the old tapes and stories that are sometimes deeply embedded in the subconscious.

Feeling safe to express and integrate these emotions ultimately leads to being able to live life in a more open and expansive state.

Over-stimulation as a result of the fast pace of life in the city means that most city dwellers are operating on FFF and running around in a state of high anxiety. Breathing then comes from the chest which requires the use of accessory muscles in the neck and shoulders resulting in chronic neck and shoulder tension. This is a physiological response to a threat of danger. When we cannot bring conscious awareness to the breath, we may be living in a constant state of anxiety and reacting from fear-based emotions; essentially, we are always ready to react rather than respond. It doesn't take much for someone in this state to be tipped over the edge and react to something trivial. Take road rage for example. I drive around London a lot and have witnessed many of these types of incidences. A driver cuts in front of a car, the car behind beeps their horn in rage and shouts profanity out of the window at the offender. In some cases, I have seen drivers get out of their car and threaten the 'offender'.

### *Transformational Breath®*
Transformational Breath® (founded by Judith Kravitz in the late '70s) is a conscious, connected breathing technique, meaning there is no pause between the inhale and exhale. It differs to pranayama and yogic breathing in that it is done through an open mouth. This helps to open up the entire respiratory system, sending energy to every physiological system in the body. When working with a trained facilitator they will use body mapping, applying pressure to certain points on the body to help open the breath and get if flowing more freely. I have seen miracles happen using Transformational Breath®, in that it can quickly access the subconscious mind through a continuous connected breath. It can also help integrate past trauma and negative emotions that have been suppressed and repressed. Remember, when we experience pain, we hold the breath. It has been said that a Transformational Breath® session is the equivalent to two years of psychotherapy.

While working on a retreat, I met a young girl, Maiya, who was 20 years old. She had chronic fatigue syndrome and debilitating chronic pain. She'd been to see numerous specialists including the 'best' in Harley Street. After two hours working with diaphragm release, specific activation points in the body that help downregulate the autonomic nervous system, diaphragmatic breathing and the connected breath, she got up with no pain whatsoever and no fatigue for the first time in a long time! The pain and fatigue was gone for a few months, and she was able to do things that many of us take for granted, such as walking the dog and washing her hair. We continue to work together, along with my partner Warren Williams, who has been providing mental, emotional and spiritual coaching. Here Maiya shares her story:

> *I didn't believe in miracles before Fran came into my life but August 2018 is the month that will forever hold a special place in my heart. I was 20, living with at times severe, chronic fatigue which left me bed-bound for weeks at a time. I also had complex regional pain syndrome in my hands, feet and knees that left me with excruciating, deep, burning pain, hot red blotches and stone cold blue patches all over my skin. Any contact with the floor or putting my weight through my limbs resulted in instant swelling and pain. Looking back, I don't know how I pushed through each day. I was desperate to do everything I could to help myself as the fatigue struck just before I was going to university to study dance, but no one knew how to help.*

> *I visited numerous doctors some of whom told me, 'I do not want to see you until you are more accepting that this is your new life now.' Some advised me to spend three months in bed not moving, just sleeping so I'd be 'less tired.' When you don't know any different, you trust in this advice (which you pay for) and you hope and pray it works. Of course, it didn't. I was oscillating between spending a few weeks in bed and a week being half-normal. Washing my hair was only possible with a rest day either side. I had no knowledge of the power of my own breath or the power that lays in the body to heal itself.*

> *After a year, I met Fran. Fran's intuition never fails, and she says she knew before meeting me she was going to help me. Looking back, I became unusually nervous before meeting her, as if I knew there was*

*going to be a big transformation. By the time I stepped into my first breath session, I was needing help to stay standing if I wanted to go for a walk. The power of my own breath blew me away within moments. My body was buzzing, and I was feeling sensations I couldn't explain. Fran is the most beautiful facilitator who holds space so well and for a first time breather this is exactly what I needed. After 2 hours, I hadn't processed what had just happened at all but I sat up and I remember just looking at Fran and crying. I could feel my body had shifted into this 'freed' state, something I couldn't put into words. The beautiful surroundings we were in looked 50% brighter. I kept closing my eyes and asking, "What's going on? Everything's changed colour." My perception of the world instantly shifted!*

*However, it didn't stop there and the second I stood up, for the first time in four years, I had no pain, no colour change, no swelling and I felt like I was in a new body. I felt like I could smile — and it was different — a smile that just radiated from within. I am a contemporary dancer and the first thing I wanted to do was dance. Any form of dance previously made me physically sick and exhausted more than I can put into words — not any more. I felt like I could fly, and never stop! It was the most beautifully breath taking moment to date. That night when I was back in Fran's restorative yoga class, I opened my tearful eyes and whispered to Fran "I can breathe!" Who knew I'd spent 20 years not breathing properly?*

*One of the greatest gifts Fran and the power of my breath has taught me is my ability to shift my perspective of the world. Fran and breathwork has taught me to rename the chronic fatigue to adrenal fatigue — something that can be healed when you change your lifestyle, thoughts and emotions. Chronic fatigue Syndrome or ME (myalgic encephalomyelitis) is a lifelong condition that doesn't have a cure, whereas adrenal fatigue most definitely has.*

*Through the continuous support from Fran and Warren teaching me how to cultivate my life force with a range of energy building exercises, grounding work, mental, emotional and spiritual coaching, I am eternally grateful that I have been able to heal this part of me and now have greater energy than I've had in years. Severe adrenal fatigue is fortunately a thing of the past. I can work towards living the life I dream every single day.*

*Fran, words will never come close to the deep gratitude I feel for the gift you gave me and continue to still give me. I never knew the power of my own body, my own breath, until this very moment. I never believed in miracles before I met you but there is no doubting you are mine. Without you there would be no me. Thank you for saving my life!'* — Maiya Leeke, 22, contemporary dancer

Through my training as a Transformational Breath® facilitator, I am trained to read different breathing patterns through a breath analysis. Often the way that we breathe links to how we are dealing with life. Ask yourself, 'Is life flowing for me?' or 'Am I stuck?' Is your breath flowing? Are you always trying to hold everything together? Are you someone who holds your body in tight, constantly bracing and holding yourself together? That was me.

For those of us coming from a fitness background, it's standard to hold 'everything in tight' or 'hold the abs in'. Women frequently suck or hold the belly in to appear slimmer and flatten the stomach. Men may brace and contract their abdomen to appear strong and tough. This creates an inverted breathing pattern where the belly draws in while inhaling, resulting in the diaphragm shutting down and an over-recruitment of the muscles of the neck and shoulders. The delivery of blood with oxygen and nutrients to the abdominal organs is compromised leading to digestive, reproductive and menstrual problems. Restoring optimal breathing mechanics is often overlooked by doctors and therapists, yet helps alleviate many common ailments. Excessive isolative training of the abdomen and abdominal tone can also create an inverted breathing pattern. No point having a six-pack if your diaphragm is not moving and stuck.

I remember, years ago my abdominals used to be rock solid from training. Whilst on a training course in abdominal massage, when it was my turn to have massage on the abdomen, my belly felt so tight. It was then that I had a realisation that my guts and stomach were so 'locked up'. I was quite proud of my rock-hard abs at the time, but I remember the teacher saying you can be strong and have tone, but the tissue should be soft and pliable. That's when it really hit me; that I was completely locked up around the guts and stomach, I was constantly bracing and holding myself in tight as a defence mechanism without even realising that I was. In a way I was bracing myself against life, which is exhausting in itself; no wonder I kept hitting the edge of burnout. Nevertheless, after having abdominal massage, I felt calmer, more peaceful and more connected to myself than ever before. That was a pivotal moment for me in my training and my path of holistic well-being.

*'When you breathe correctly, you create more mental-emotional stability in your body and unload tension within the viscera so the organ systems become healthier.'* — Ashley Mazurek, CHEK practitioner and faculty

### Box Breathing

Box breathing is a simple technique used by the Navy Seals in highly stressed situations. It is a great and effective technique to help keep calm and control of your thoughts when under stress. It's great for anxiety and as a sleep aid.

Simply:

1.  Inhale for four seconds
2.  Hold the breath for four seconds
3.  Exhale for four seconds
4.  Hold your lungs empty for four seconds

Repeat for six rounds and up to as many rounds as you like. However, do not do this if you are pregnant or think you might be.

### Health Bank Deposits

✓ Observe where your breath is. Is it more in the chest or the belly?

✓ Take ten deep abdominal breaths in and out through the nose

✓ Try the box breath

## An Attitude Of Gratitude

Cultivating an attitude of gratitude is one of the highest vibrational states you can be in.

*'Something as simple as moving into an elevated state of love, joy or gratitude for five to ten minutes a day can produce significant epigenetic changes in our health and bodies.'* — Dr Joe Dispenza

Professor of Psychology at the University of California, Robert A. Emmons, says:

*'The practice of gratitude can have dramatic and lasting effects in a person's life. Gratitude blocks toxic emotions, such as envy, resentment, regret and depression, which can destroy our happiness'.*

It's impossible to feel envious and grateful at the same time. I've kept a gratitude journal for years, writing down three to five things a day that I am thankful for. It's heart-warming to look back on my past journals over the years and reflect upon memories that I was grateful for years ago. You can begin today. Buy yourself a beautiful notebook and write three to five things you are thankful for each morning / evening. I like to do it in the evening, before bed, because it helps to clear my head and let go of any tension I'm holding onto from the day. It also helps me to have a truly restful sleep, ending my day in thanks and appreciation. You are more likely to wake up in the emotional state you went to bed in. I tell my clients if they go to bed pissed off, they are more likely to wake up feeling pissed off. Change your emotional state simply through having an attitude of gratitude. There are now gratitude apps too such as *Grateful: A Gratitude Journal, Gratitude — Happiness Journal and Happyfeed — Gratitude Journal* that you can download onto your device. They allow you to create pictures of the things you are grateful for. This can make a lovely photo diary to look back on.

Once every few weeks, I'll go on a rampage of appreciation, putting pen to paper and writing up to 50 things I'm thankful for. It immediately shifts my mindset and I feel so abundant. I highly recommend doing this and really bathing in the emotions and the feeling of gratitude for everything on your list. The exercise serves so many purposes and is especially great when you are feeling low. I've found it a powerful exercise in situations and circumstances that perhaps hadn't turned out as I had wanted at the time. It helps to free the energetic charge around situations that were not always in my control, like a job opportunity or a relationship not working out. You then realise that in every situation there is always a lesson or a blessing.

Start with the small things. For example:

I am thankful for food in the fridge.

I am thankful for a roof over my head.

I am thankful for the clothes on my back.

There are so many people in the world who go without the simple things we may take for granted. You are richer than 75% of the world if you have a roof over your head and a place to sleep, food in your fridge and clothes on your back. If you are reading this book, you are more fortunate than the *billion* people in the world who cannot read at all.

### Gratitude Exercise

Write down ten things / people / places / experiences / circumstances you are thankful for today and *feel* the appreciation and gratitude flood into your heart and body, lighting up every cell. Really bathe in the *feeling* of gratitude.

1. I am so thankful for *Ciara's friendship*
2. I am so thankful for *going to Shore Clair*
3. I am so thankful for *a tasty dinner*
4. I am so thankful for *new toiletries*
5. I am so thankful for *coffee w/ mum*
6. I am so thankful for *football + food w/ family*
7. I am so thankful for *ben cleaning his shoes*
8. I am so thankful for *my new weather Anna*
9. I am so thankful for *my lovely pyjamas*
10. I am so thankful for *marta coming tomorrow*

### Health Bank Deposits

✓ Buy a beautiful journal to use for writing down the things you are grateful for. Write three to five things / people / places / experiences / circumstances that you are grateful for each morning / evening

✓ Bathe in the *feeling* of gratitude; being in a state of gratitude blocks toxic emotions

✓ Every now and again, go on a rampage of appreciation

✓ Do the gratitude exercise, writing down ten things you are grateful for.

## Meditation

Meditation has been a game-changer for me. It helps me to start my day grounded and calm for the day ahead. When I first started, like most people, I found it really hard; my mind was so active and I couldn't relax, squinting with one eye open to check on the time and see how long I had been meditating for. Meditation has a cumulative effect and now I feel it when I don't do it.

I first went along a few times to a beautiful Buddhist centre in West London where the meditation sessions were led by a monk. I always found a deep sense of peace afterwards; however, continuing with it myself on my own was really challenging. My mind was too active, running away in all directions with my 'To do' list. I resumed in 2014 when I started yoga teacher training in India. We would do 30 minutes of group meditation every evening and it was wonderful to hear the soothing sounds of nature in the open yoga shala even with the mosquitoes biting us. I felt so peaceful, relaxed, grounded and calm. After training, I spent two months there and some time in an ashram in Kerala. It was therefore easy to meditate every day.

I returned to London feeling amazing. I'd slowed down so much, and people commented on how different I looked. The feeling stayed with me for a few months and during that time, I felt like a rooted tree standing strong among the chaos. The contrast between Kerala and its famous still backwaters and beach life and the fast pace of the city was stark. Everyone around me was stressed and I could feel they were like pressure cookers ready to explode. At the time I was also a personal trainer in a gym that was loud, cluttered and at times quite hectic — not exactly a zen space. The mistake I made was that because I felt so good and grounded, my meditation practice went out of the window. Guess what? It wasn't long before the roots of my tree withered and I was once again swept up into the fast-moving energy of London.

What I've learnt is that it's easy to be still in the mountains or on a retreat and meditate when there are no distractions. The real test is maintaining that when you are busy, when there is chaos all around you, when life is fast-paced, when you have relationship problems, financial stress and your kids are fighting. Can you be grounded and resilient among the chaos and during the storm? No matter what is going on around you, true spiritual practice is finding inner peace and being centred amongst the chaos. It took me a while to get that, but eventually I did. It takes time, practice and discipline, but it's fundamental in becoming the master of your reality. I will go into this more when I talk about creating a morning ritual where you create habits that soon become your default setting.

In 2015, a few different people recommended Vedic meditation to me. I ended up at Will Williams Meditation in London (now known as Beeja Meditation). Through Will Williams, I learnt about the science of meditation, the effect it has on the body and hormonal system and how repeating a mantra specific to you helps to regulate the frequency at which your nervous system vibrates. I was fascinated. The practice takes 20 minutes, twice a day. Understanding more about the benefits and science behind meditation motivated me to keep it up as a daily practice. So, what is the science behind meditation?

### The Science and Benefits of Meditation
Research has shown meditation to be associated with less stress, depression, anxiety, pain, insomnia and an increased quality of life. It actually changes your brain! *Lazar et al* (2005) found that meditation was associated with more grey matter in the frontal cortex of the brain, the area associated with memory and executive decision-making. In another study by *Hölzel et al* (2011), a mindfulness-based stress reduction programme was carried out over eight weeks with 16 beginner meditators. MRI scans found that the brain volume increased in five different regions of the subjects. The primary difference was found in the posterior cingulate which is involved in mind-wandering and self-relevance. Regions of the brain involved in learning, cognition, memory, emotional regulation, empathy and

compassion were found to have increased in volume too. Interestingly, the amygdala, associated with the fight and flight was found to shrink, which is great for anxiety, fear and stress.

### Meditation Exercise

Meditation is not about completely emptying the mind or having absence of thoughts, but simply quieting the mind and becoming unattached to the thoughts that do come through. In busy modern life today, it is extremely challenging to stop the stream of mind chatter. If you are new to meditation, start with just a few minutes a day. Find a comfortable place to sit down with your back supported against something. Close your eyes and take a deep breath in through your nose and a sigh out through your mouth. Repeat two more times. Stretch the jaw open a few times and roll the shoulders back, releasing any tension. Feel yourself sitting deep into your seat, into your hips and pelvis where your power centre lies.

Now, imagine yourself standing by a stream as you listen to the sounds of nature around you and the soothing sound of a freshwater stream. Let any thoughts coming through float by and down the stream as you simply observe them passing without attaching to them. Come back to your breath and to your centre. Do this for five minutes to begin with and then gradually increase by a few minutes each week, building up to 20 minutes. You will find the mind chatter gets less and less, creating space to be still. It is in the stillness that you access your intuition, connect to your higher self and allow creative ideas to flow through.

It's a practice that takes discipline and time. Set the same time each day to meditate so that it becomes a habit and then a daily practice. I now meditate every morning, no matter what time I need to get up. It sets me up for a day of working with clients or delivering workshops. It helps me to be grounded and relaxed. If I miss my session for a few days (which is rare these days), I definitely feel the difference as I'm more impatient, angsty and easily irritated.

### *Health Bank Deposits*

✓ Meditate at the same time each day

✓ Start with just a few minutes and build up to 20 minutes at a time

✓ Be disciplined and dedicated to your daily practice so that it becomes a habit

✓ If your mind is very busy, try a walking meditation or my **Working In** program on page 84. Take a walk in nature, turn your phone off and observe the beautiful environment around you. In London, we're so fortunate to have many beautiful green open spaces available to the public so take advantage of them.

# PART 2

# The Body

## Sleep And Circadian Rhythms

The power and healing benefits of sleep cannot be underestimated. In the last few years there has been a lot of research into the land of nod. There are books on sleep and even sleep retreats. It's necessary as we are now in a global crisis of sleep-deprived humans operating on autopilot and fuelled by caffeine and stimulants. Some companies even provide beds in the office now so that you can work long hours and not even go home because you have the privilege of 'sleeping in the office'. As a holistic lifestyle coach, I was taught about being in flow with the circadian rhythms and have been teaching my clients about it ever since. The circadian rhythm is like a 24-hour internal body clock that regulates the sleep / wake cycle and all other biological rhythms.

Sleep should be a number-one priority. It's the most cost-effective medicine there is. Lack of sleep and poor sleep rhythms upset the hormonal rhythms, creating a host of health ailments such as muscle aches and pains, headaches, adrenal fatigue, joint pain, inflammation, bacterial and fungal infections, a lowered immune system and even weight gain. For thousands of years we've lived in tune with the rhythms of nature and the light and dark cycles of day and night. The human body is incredibly intelligent, releasing specific hormones such as cortisol in accordance with these cycles. When light hits the skin or eyes, whether natural or artificial, your brain and hormonal system thinks it's daytime.

*'Our physiology is still the same as our ancient sun driven ancestors; we're simply packaged in fancy clothes, drive cars and use lots of electronic gadgets.'* — Paul Chek

We're still hard-wired to be in sync with this natural rhythm and it has been witnessed in wildlife just how influential light is over the physiology. During solar eclipses, animals have gone to sleep thinking it's night-time only to wake up soon after the eclipse passes confused and dazed. This was particularly noted at the solar eclipse on 11 August, 1999.

Most cities are buzzing 24 hours a day. That can be fun and exciting with endless attractions, things to do and places to eat. However, it's not optimal for health in the long-term. If you live on a street with bright street lamps streaming into your bedroom, this will affect the quality of your sleep. I lived in a basement flat in London for a few years where my bedroom faced the street; the light from the lamp post streaming in made my sleep light and restless. A study conducted by Ohayon and Milesi in 2016, showed outdoor night-time street lighting to be associated with greater dissatisfaction with sleep quality and/or quantity and a greater likelihood of a diagnostic profile congruent with a circadian rhythm disorder. The solution? Blackout blinds or curtains.

### Tech Hangover

In 2012, the American Medical Association's Council on Science and Public Health stated that: 'Exposure to excessive light at night, including extended use of various electronic media, can disrupt sleep or exacerbate sleep disorders.'[9]

Bright lights, TV screens and blue light from computers, phones and screens also trick the brain and hormonal system into thinking it's daytime, stimulating the release of cortisol. I certainly notice a significant difference when I have been on my devices late at night. My sleep is not as deep or restful and I wake up feeling groggy — the tech hangover.

A study by Mariana Figueiro and her team at the Lighting Research Center at Rensselaer Polytechnic Institute in Troy, New York, discovered that night-time release of melatonin was significantly suppressed with just two hours of computer screen time before bed (*Wood et al*, 2012). It can take hours to clear cortisol from the bloodstream, inhibiting the release of melatonin and growth hormones, cutting into the immune system's valuable repair time. Ideally, you should stop any screen time two hours before bed. We do live in a busy technological world, and sometimes this is not always possible; see below some of my sleep hacks to get around this when it is not always possible.

---

9   American Medical Association's Council on Science and Public Health (2012) — AMA Report of the Council of Science and Public Health, p12

When working with some of my clients that had sleep issues, the number-one reason for this was their phones — either sleeping with their phone switched on by their bed, charging their phone close to the bed and browsing on their devices late at night. Once they stopped all these practices, or even just put their phone on airplane mode, their sleep improved dramatically. It has been reported that we get a dopamine hit every time a notification comes through on our phone, like a text from a loved one or a social media like.[10] Dopamine is a brain chemical that keeps us seeking more of this hit as it makes us feel good. Having phones on in the bedroom while you sleep is a distraction. So, put your phone on airplane mode as far away from your bed as possible or, better still, completely out of the bedroom to avoid the late-night scrolling temptation. That midnight email really can wait. Use a natural wake-up light alarm instead of relying on your phone alarm. Invest in some blue light-blocking glasses or use the app FLUX on your devices to limit blue light emittance. A dim red light at night is the least disruptive to the circadian rhythm. Himalayan salt lamps are great to use in the home also, with their soft, warming pink lighting, and are very reasonably priced.

A 2008 study published by the Massachusetts Institute of Technology's Progress in Electromagnetic Research Symposium, sponsored by the mobile phone companies themselves, found that radiation from mobile phone usage before bed delayed and reduced sleep, causing headaches and confusion.[11] It affected the quality of sleep by taking longer for the subjects to reach the deeper stages of sleep and spend less time there. This disrupted the vital growth and repair cycle necessary to repair damage suffered during the day. If children and teenagers don't get enough quality sleep they can develop mood and personality changes, attention deficit hyperactivity disorder (ADHD)-like symptoms, depression, lack of concentration

---

10 Has dopamine got us hooked on tech (2018) — www.theguardian.com/technology/2018/mar/04/has-dopamine-got-us-hooked-on-tech-facebook-apps-addiction

11 Mobile phone radiation wrecks your sleep by Geoffrey Lean, Environment Editor (2008) — www.independent.co.uk/life-style/health-and-families/health-news/mobile-phone-radiation-wrecks-your-sleep-771262.html

and poor performance. Switch off your Wi-Fi hub at night for the same reasons. The above results are from a study carried out over ten years ago; it's frightening to think what future studies will show as smartphones and devices become more advanced.

### Hormones and Sleep

When the stress hormone cortisol is released it prepares you for action and movement. As discussed in Part One not all stress is bad; we need some to give us our get up and go, move and be productive. If you are in sync with your circadian rhythms, then first thing in the morning as the sun rises the body produces a surge of cortisol, because you are meant to wake up feeling refreshed and in action mode. The rhythm of cortisol release fluctuates through the day, remaining high to midday to support daily activities. It naturally starts to taper off in the afternoon, dropping significantly as the sun goes down. This is the ideal time to start winding down from your day. It's a reason why many people crave the 3pm coffee or sugar hit to get some stimulation. At this time, I encourage clients to have a fat snack like an avocado with lemon and Himalayan salt, a handful of walnuts and berries, a fat bomb (see page 74 for recipe) or a greens powder mixed with coconut water. You'll get some energy without the adrenal and insulin spike that comes with the coffee and sugar, which can then affect your quality of sleep.

As the sun goes down, cortisol levels decrease and growth and repair hormones are released. The latter cannot be released though if cortisol levels remain high. Therefore it's a bad idea to do any intense training or exercise late in the evening. I've experienced this first-hand. In my early 20s, I used to teach spin classes and train clients most evenings, working in gyms with bright lights, TV screens and loud music until up to 10 o'clock at night. I'd get home buzzing, wired and tired, but couldn't switch off because my nervous system was so stimulated. Eventually I was exhausted so I stopped training clients and doing any intense physical activity in the evening. It's one of the reasons I burnt out and lost alignment with my number one core value of health. This was a familiar story for many other fitness professionals I knew. We would be doing a lot of physical activity yet struggle to lose weight and feel 'inflamed'. The only activities I recommend late in the evening are restorative practices like Tai Chi, Qigong, yoga, dancing and sex.

We are humans designed to bounce back from intermittent stress, and so a late night or two every now and again is fine, but continuously can create chronic health problems in the long-term. The ideal time to go to sleep is 10 – 10:30pm. Between 10pm – 2am, growth and repair hormones are released which are vital for physical repair and even more important if you are an athlete. From 2 – 6am, mental repair takes place, when the active brain neurons rest and the supportive glial cells clean up the toxins and debris produced by the neurons. The ideal amount of sleep is seven to nine hours but there is a small percentage of people who are genetically different and don't need as much. Most of us do though. If you want to improve physical, emotional, brain and neurological health, get to bed early.

### Lose Weight By Sleeping

Research led by Dr Eve Van Cauter into the relationship between sleep disturbances, circadian dysregulation, obesity and diabetes in the past two decades shows that sleep loss and poor sleep quality were significant risk factors for weight gain and abnormal blood glucose tolerance, increasing the risk of diabetes (*Knutson and Cauter, 2015*). Altered levels of hormones related to hunger and appetite, such as leptin and ghrelin, occurred in sleep-deprived individuals. Leptin is a hormone that lets you know when you are satiated and full, while ghrelin is known as the 'hunger hormone' that stimulates appetite. A study published in the *Journal of Sleep Research* by *Schmid et al* (2008) found a single night of sleep deprivation increased ghrelin levels and feelings of hunger in normal-weight, healthy men, increasing the risk of weight gain and obesity.

Conclusion? A good night's sleep is important for weight control.

### Let's Talk About Sex Baby

Earlier, we talked about avoiding intense physical activity late in the evening. Now I know some of you will be thinking, 'Well? What about sex, that's physical?' Yes, sex is physical. However, it comes with a host of benefits that improve your sleep. Research has shown that a cocktail of chemicals are released during orgasm in both men and women. These include oxytocin, serotonin and norepinephrine. So, don't worry about skipping that late night activity! Oxytocin, the love hormone that promotes bonding between two people when they are engaged intimately, has a calming influence that counters the effects of cortisol and helps induce sleep. Serotonin, the body's powerful anti-stress neurotransmitter, has been shown to be critical in maintaining normal sleep-wake cycles, according to research published in the *Journal of Progress in Neurobiology* by *Portas et al* (2000). Norepinephrine helps regulate normal sleep-wake cycles and helps with the synthesis of melatonin. It plays an important role in balancing the overall stress response in the body.

### Creating a Wind-Down Routine

‣ Switch off electronics, ideally two hours before bed

‣ Read a book

‣ Write in your gratitude journal — helps you switch off from the action of the day and bathe in the feeling of gratitude

‣ Have a Himalayan / Epsom salt / magnesium warm bath. Magnesium helps with sleep and is depleted in times of stress

‣ Avoid eating at least two hours before bed to allow complete digestion

‣ Avoid caffeine after lunch

‣ On Apple devices, you can go to settings and change display and brightness to night shift; it sets a soft orange tone (like sunset) on your device and reduces blue light which makes your brain think it's daytime (blue sky)

‣ Invest in some blue light-blocking glasses if on devices in the evening

Create a room sanctuary. Your bedroom should be for sleep and sex only. If you work from the day in your bedroom and use your bedroom as an office, you are more likely to be thinking about work as you go to bed and are less likely to switch off. Creating a warm safe environment in your bedroom is highly conducive to sleep.

## *Tip*

For those with young children and particularly mothers, getting a few hours of unbroken sleep would be bliss! Most parents with young children are sleep-deprived. A study by *Hoekzema et al* (2017) looked at brain scans of women during pregnancy soon after giving birth and two years later. They found that the volume of grey matter in the brain that was associated with social interactions and 'theory of mind' tasks was significantly reduced up to two years after giving birth for first-time mothers. Hence the term 'baby brain'. I recommend to my clients with young babies and children to:

- Take naps when your baby takes a nap. Power naps for 20 minutes listening to binaural beats on headphones have been shown to bring the brainwaves into a more restorative state in a short period of time.
- Follow my self-care practices outlined in this book, particularly around food and work in exercises to raise your vitality as high as you can while sleep is compromised.

## *Night Shifters*

Night shift work is not ideal and, in the long run, is detrimental to health. If it cannot be avoided, the best thing to do is to keep your physiology in a regular rhythm, eating your meals, going to bed and waking up at the same time each day until you can transition to working in a way that is more supportive to your physiology. Meditation and power naps are also beneficial. Just 20 minutes of each can have the benefits of the deepest state of sleep. Varying shifts within the week plays havoc with the circadian and hormonal rhythms and is not sustainable for long-term health. Sadly, most people working like this usually eventually burn out.

### Health Bank Deposits

✓ Have a wind-down routine

✓ Use blackout blinds or curtains in the bedroom

✓ Do not charge your phone by your bed

✓ Remove electronic gadgets from your bedroom

✓ Turn off your Wi-Fi hub at night if you have access to it

✓ Turn phone on airplane mode and even leave it out of the bedroom to avoid distractions and midnight scrolling

✓ Remove or put away any work from your day

✓ Wake up to a soothing alarm clock like a natural wake-up light or one that has the sound of the morning birds

✓ Use bed sheets made from natural materials such as cotton, linen, hemp or silk

✓ Add some flora and fauna — green plants are great for oxygenating the air

✓ Dim lights and use soft lighting like Himalayan salt lamps that emit soft pink warming light in the evening

✓ Light non-toxic candles in the evening (remember blow them out before sleeping)

# Food As Nature Intended

*'Let food be thy medicine and medicine be thy food.'* — Hippocrates

I *love* food.

I'm a foodie and I absolutely love food that's wholesome, real, unprocessed and that nourishes my mind, body and soul. Food and what you eat is high up on the list of optimum self-care. However, there is so much information out there on what to eat, what not to eat, as well as countless diets to subscribe to. My advice is to keep it simple:

- ▸ Eat as nature intended
- ▸ Connect to what your body really wants — eat intuitively
- ▸ Buy the highest quality food you can afford
- ▸ Differentiate between food and non-food

Unfortunately, today's food is so depleted. Supermarket fruits and vegetables are transported halfway across the world, and by the time they get to us they contain very little nutritional value. Most fruits, vegetables and grains are laden with harmful chemical pesticides, herbicides and fungicides that end up in our bodies. Commercially-farmed meats come from animals that are raised consuming unnatural foods (often pesticide-sprayed grains), injected with growth hormones and antibiotics and living in confined spaces. Genetically modified (GM) foods have entered the food industry and no one knows the long-term health implications of these unnatural, altered foods that go against Mother Nature. GM foods are not required to prove their safety before they are sold; in essence we are human guinea pigs.

In an ideal world we'd be living off the land, growing our own organic fruits and vegetables in our backyard and rearing our own livestock that roam the land under plenty of daylight. However, in the city, it's rare to even have garden space these days. Nevertheless, we are not helpless when it comes to eating the best we can. Your health is your wealth and it's important to know where your food is coming from; you can still make a conscious effort to consume as much high-quality foods as you can afford for yourself and your family.

## Organic

My parents' and grandparents' generation grew up on natural foods so by default most food was organic. They cooked fresh from scratch and there was little chance of eating processed and packaged 'non-foods'. They simply ate food as nature intended. It saddens me that organic food (which is food in its natural state without being sprayed with harmful chemicals, hormone-injected meats and genetically modified foods) is the exception and not the rule. How has it become normal to consume artificial foods? No wonder there is such a rise in cancers, heart disease, diabetes and obesity. Unfortunately big food companies and commercial farms are not interested in your health, but profit, and so their practices are driven by the latter.

*'The food industry employs teams of scientists to improve the "mouthfeel" of fake processed food and maximise food cravings.'* — Dr Mercola

It really is down to *you* to go against the grain and take *your* health in *your* own hands so as not to become another statistic.

## What Does Organic Even Mean?

Under European law, organic means produced with natural substances and processes. This means much lower levels of pesticides are used, as are manufactured herbicides, artificial colours, preservatives or genetically modified foods. For animals reared for meat, drugs, antibiotics and wormers are not routinely used. Food is as it should be.

Did you know that almost 300 pesticides are routinely used in non-organic farming? Government testing in the UK found pesticide residue in 47 per cent of British food, and farm animals account for almost two-thirds of all antibiotic use in the European Union! Certified organic farmers are permitted to use up to 20 pesticides derived from natural ingredients like citronella. Organic is not only better for your health but for the entire planet, helping to reduce water and soil contamination from synthetic and petroleum-based fertilisers and cut greenhouse gas emissions.

For more information, I highly recommend checking out www.soilassociation.org

## *Glyphosate*

The use of glyphosate, one of the most widely used herbicides worldwide, originally created by US agrochemical company Monsanto, has increased 400 per cent in UK farming over the last 20 years. It has been found in over 60 per cent of wholemeal bread samples tested by the Department of Environment Food and Rural Affairs (DEFRA)[12] and is now present everywhere in the food chain including water. In 2015, 17 experts from 11 different countries met at the International Agency for Research on Cancer (IARC) to review the published evidence on the carcinogenicity of glyphosate[13]. Glyphosate was declared as a 'probable carcinogen', meaning there is sufficient evidence of causing cancer on lab animals but limited evidence in humans (mainly because there have been very few studies on humans as it would be unethical). Professor Christopher Portier, one of the co-authors of the IARC report, reiterated the IARC's conclusions, stating: "Glyphosate is definitely genotoxic. There is no doubt in my mind".[14] Definitely genotoxic meaning to cause cell mutations and DNA damage.

Roundup®, the commercial name for a glyphosate-based herbicide, was found to contain other chemicals 125 times more toxic when mixed together than glyphosate alone (*Mesnage et al, 2014*). Though Monsanto and US regulatory agencies of course claim glyphosate does not bio-accumulate in the organs and bones, a study in 2014 published in the *Journal of Environmental and Analytical Toxicology* found glyphosate residues in multiple organs of slaughtered cows (*Krüger et al, 2014*). In this same study glyphosate was significantly higher in humans fed conventional food than those predominantly fed with organic food. Chronically ill humans had significantly higher residues in their urine. Most recently, 2019 testing and analysis performed by Anresco laboratories, San Francisco, an FDA-registered laboratory, found

---

12 Department of Environment Food and Rural Affairs — https://rio.jrc.ec.europa.eu/en/organisations/department-environment-food-and-rural-affairs-defra
13 International Agency for Research on Cancer (2015) — 'IARC Monograph on Glyphosate' www.iarc.fr/featured-news/media-centre-iarc-news-glyphosate/
14 Monsato's Roundup (Glyphosate) damages DNA says World Health Organization Expert (2015) — https://www.globalresearch.ca/monsantos-roundup-glyphosate-damages-dna-says-world-health-organisation-expert/5462631

shockingly high levels of glyphosate in the cereal Cheerios® — a cereal for children.[15]

The likelihood of this herbicide being carcinogenic, and without knowing the long-term effects and implications on human health and the generations to come, is enough of a deterrent for me. We really are playing with life here, and if you want to thrive and experience vibrant health and vitality, then it starts with eating as nature intended, i.e., food that has not been heavily sprayed and contaminated with chemicals. Simply search in google 'person spraying pesticides' and you will see in every image someone covered head to toe in protective gear. If it's harmful to the person spraying the chemicals, surely it is harmful to ingest food covered with it.

A recent toxicology report published in 2018 by *Defarge et al* identified other heavy metals such as arsenic, chromium, cobalt, lead and nickel known as endocrine disruptors in pesticide formulations. The pesticide dichlorodiphenyltrichloroethane (DDT) was widely used for insect control on crops and livestock for three decades before being banned in 1972 in the US. It has been shown to affect the nervous system, accumulate in fatty tissue, be acutely toxic to animals and humans if eaten and cause sterility, birth defects and reproductive issues in lab mice. It is labelled as being carcinogenic and is still used in South America, Asia and Africa to control malaria and other diseases. Is it going to be another 30 years before it is deemed unsafe to use glyphosate on food? Will it be too late by then?

Recent research studies by Średnicka-Tober in 2016 at Newcastle University published in the *British Journal of Nutrition*, and the largest study of its kind found:

- ▸ Non-organic fruit to have the highest pesticide frequency (75%) compared with non-organic vegetables (32%) and non-organic, crop-based processed foods (45%)

---

15 Glyphosate: Unsafe on any plate (2019) Report by Food Democracy Now and The Detox Project — s3.amazonaws.com/media.fooddemocracynow.org/images/FDN_ Glyphosate_FoodTesting_Report_p2016.pdf

- ▸ 48% lower concentrations of the toxic heavy metal cadmium detected in organic crops (*Barański et al, 2014*)
- ▸ Up to 69% more anti-oxidants in organic than non-organic food
- ▸ 50% more beneficial omega-3-fatty acids in organic milk and meat than non-organic versions
- ▸ Organic milk and dairy contained 39% more conjugated linolenic acid (CLA) that has been shown to have great benefits for cardiovascular health, protect against certain cancers, diabetes and obesity

The results speak for themselves.

### But I Can't Afford Organic

While I appreciate organic does usually cost more sometimes, given the research and statistics above, I invite you to ask — 'can you afford not to? If your health is a priority, the quality of food you choose to eat must also be a priority. It may mean cutting back on other things, such as your meat intake and having only high-quality animal products every now and again rather than daily. It could mean cutting back on packaged and processed foods that are nutritionally low and replacing with higher-quality, nutritionally dense fruits, vegetables and herbs. You'll find you won't feel the need to eat as much as you are getting better-quality nutrients.

Organic certification is a lengthy and very expensive process for farmers, especially independent, small farms. Many of them are passionate about their farming practices and adhere to organic and biodynamic practices but can't afford the certification price tag. I've found the best produce at local farmers' markets; the meat and produce often tastes much better than that of supermarket 'certified organic'. Check out www.lfm.org.uk for a list of farmers' markets in London and how the produce is grown / raised. Go in the last hour when you are sure to get more deals as stallholders want to get rid of their produce. There are many pick-your-own farms which are a great way for children to connect with where their food is coming from.

There are food delivery boxes such as Abel & Cole and Riverford (see recommended resources at the back) where all the produce adheres to organic practices. You can taste the difference. In London, there are so many amazing home food delivery schemes of produce straight from the farm that have organic practices and care about sustainability and the health of our planet.

## Tips

### Ask for the cheaper cuts of meat

I recommend going to a good butcher or local farmers' market and asking for the cheaper cuts of meat — beef skirt, flank, bavette or brisket. Ask for a chicken carcass / beef bones. They may even give it to you for free, or for a couple of pounds, and you can make a highly nutritious and delicious, gut-healing bone broth that will last you a while (depending on how many you are feeding; see my recipe on page 73).

### Grill non-organic food

If cooking non-organic meats and fish, grill them on a rack and allow the fat to drip down. Toxins store in fat so if you drain as much fat off as you can, you consume less toxins.

## The Dirty Dozen

The Environmental Working Group (EWG) publishes an annual list of the 'Dirty Dozen' — fruits and vegetables that have the highest amounts of pesticides when grown conventionally vs organically.[16] It also prints the 'Clean Fifteen' fruits and vegetables with the least contamination and pesticide residue.

*The Dirty Dozen, 2019:*

| | | | |
|---|---|---|---|
| 1. | Strawberries | 7. | Peaches |
| 2. | Spinach | 8. | Cherries |
| 3. | Kale | 9. | Pears |
| 4. | Nectarines | 10. | Tomatoes |
| 5. | Apples | 11. | Celery |
| 6. | Grapes | 12. | Potatoes |

---

16 Shopper's guide to pesticides in produce (2019) — www.ewg.org/foodnews/

*The Clean Fifteen, 2019:*

1. Avocados
2. Sweetcorn
3. Pineapples
4. Frozen sweet peas
5. Onions
6. Papaya
7. Eggplants
8. Asparagus
9. Kiwis
10. Cabbage
11. Cauliflower
12. Cantaloupes
13. Broccoli
14. Mushrooms
15. Honeydew melon

Prioritise the Dirty Dozen to be organic and relax with the Clean Fifteen. As a general rule, any fruit or vegetable with a thicker skin will generally have a lower pesticide residue than leafy foods and berries. Always wash your fruits and vegetables before consuming. You can also use a natural veggie wash that helps remove bacteria, waxes and some pesticide residue. One I've used is Veggi-wash® (www.veggiwash.co.uk) or Bentley® organic salad, fruit and veg wash, available on Amazon or in health food stores. Make your own veggie wash by adding one to two tablespoons of apple cider vinegar to 3.5 litres of filtered, bottled or distilled water.

### Lose Weight by Eating Organic

As toxins are stored in fat, commercially-farmed produce and meat have a much higher level of toxins from pesticide residues, antibiotics and hormones. The body will hold onto fat to store these toxins and therefore protect the organs. The more natural your food is, with less residue contamination, then the body drops any excess fat as it is no longer needed to store the toxins coming in. Thus, eating organic, natural, unprocessed food as nature intended is one way to quickly stabilise body weight.

### Fat is Your Friend

For years, science and the medical industry fooled the world into believing saturated fat was bad for you and that cutting fat out of your diet would help you lose weight. The low-fat and trans-fat crazes were born — two supposedly healthier alternatives that turned out to be the most harmful for public health. Trans-fats like margarine and hydrogenated vegetable oils cannot be metabolised by the body. Weight Watchers®, Slimming World®, SlimFast® and the LighterLife® low-calorie diets were born as they packaged their highly processed, non-food products to serve to their members. Instead of improving health, heart disease, diabetes and obesity have risen in the UK and worldwide since the low-fat craze caught on. As a CHEK holistic lifestyle coach, in the early part of the millennium, I learnt about the importance of eating real, organic, wholefood produce.

Unfortunately, medical professionals receive very little specific and focussed training in nutrition and the benefits of eating well. The medical industry has been slow to catch up with the importance of the quality of foods you eat; saturated fat and cholesterol are still deemed the 'bad guys' and you are being wrongly advised to avoid them. In 1998, a study published in the *Journal of Clinical Epidemiology* examined people in 35 countries looking for a direct link between dietary fats and cardiovascular disease. None could be found. The conclusion was that 'the positive ecological correlations between national intakes of total fat and saturated fatty acids and cardiovascular mortality were absent or negative' (*Ravnskov, 1998*)

I highly recommend looking up Dr Mercola who has written various articles on the benefits of saturated fats and cholesterol for human health and performance (*Mercola, 2010; 2011*). Saturated fats, found in animal fats and tropical oils, are needed for the proper functioning of cell membranes, heart, liver, lungs, immune system, satiety, bones, hormones and genetic regulation. They make up at least 50% of the cell membranes and they give cells stiffness and integrity. Omega-3 fats are one of the most important fats you can have in your diet. They are highly anti-inflammatory. Good sources are wild salmon, coconuts, coconut oil, avocados, raw dairy, grass-fed meats, raw macadamia, almonds, pecans, seeds and organic egg yolks. It is no mistake that human breast milk, nature's finest food for a developing infant, contains 54 per cent saturated fat.

### The Great Cholesterol Con

The theory that there is a direct relationship between the amount of saturated fat and cholesterol in the diet and the incidence of coronary heart disease was first proposed by a researcher named Ancel Keys in the late '50s. Keys led the longitudinal, epidemiological study 'The Seven Countries Study,' which documented the variations in coronary heart disease risk related to diet and culture across seven countries (*Keys, 1966*). The hypothesis received great attention and became scientific fact in the medical community, even though there was no definitive research to back the theory. The public were completely misled. The famous heart surgeon, Michael DeBakey conducted a survey of 1,700 patients with hardening of the arteries and found NO relationship between the level of cholesterol in the blood and atherosclerosis (*DeBakey et al, 1964*).

Cholesterol is needed for cell membrane production, neurological function, hormone production, vitamin D and production of bile acids to help digest fat. Essentially cholesterol is needed for life. It's a precursor to all steroid sex hormones and so is necessary to produce oestrogen, testosterone, cortisone and other vital hormones. Low cholesterol has been linked to depression, stroke, violent behaviour and suicide. Lower cholesterol levels may lead to lower brain serotonin, which may lead to increased violence and aggression (*Golomb, 1998*). In a large Dutch study, chronically low cholesterol levels in men were shown to be consistently linked to a higher risk of depressive symptoms (*Steegmans et al, 2000*).

*'A high cholesterol level reflects chronic inflammation in the body. The more inflammation you have the higher the total cholesterol tends to be. Your body makes cholesterol to 'patch up' damages from this ongoing inflammation.'* — Dr Mercola

Sugar, processed foods and toxic chemicals are the major cause of inflammation, not cholesterol.

## Sugar

The average American and Englishman consumes 150 – 170 lbs of sugar per year, with an average of 42.5 teaspoons per day, compared with only four pounds of simple sugars per year 100 years ago. Naturally occurring sweetness from complex wholefood carbohydrates such as fruits and vegetables were the only available forms of sugar 400 years ago.

Sugar is stored in the liver and muscles in the form of glycogen. The liver has only a limited capacity; once full, the rest of the sugar is left circulating in the blood. Insulin, the hormone responsible for balancing blood sugar levels, responds by rapidly reducing the blood sugar, often to a very low level, known as *hypoglycaemia*, causing a blood sugar crash. The body must respond to this 'emergency' immediately. The stress hormone cortisol is secreted to release the stored glycogen from the liver and raise blood sugar levels quickly; this is often when one reaches for the coffee or sugar hit and the whole ride starts again. Insulin is a fat-storing hormone and will take this extra sugar and store it as fatty acids mostly around the belly, buttocks, hips and breasts. Before you know it, you are on a sugar rollercoaster, which is incredibly stressful for the body. This constant sugar rollercoaster, long-term, will fatigue the adrenals, create insulin resistance, increasing the risk of Type 2 diabetes, metabolic syndrome and compromising the immune system.

> Did you know...
> Wheat converts to glucose faster than any other grain, and excess glucose in the bloodstream converts to fatty acids and increases inflammation in the body. Most breakfast cereals and breads are made from wheat and are NOT a good choice for breakfast.

## Reading Labels

Ingredients are listed from the highest to the lowest proportion. Processed sugar comes in many disguises and may appear on your ingredients list as any of the below. As a guide, anything ending in '-ose' is a form of sugar. Avoid the product if any of the list over the page are listed as the first three ingredients. Be mindful of naturally occurring sugars too, such as those in fruit, dates, etc., as too much will create a blood sugar imbalance.

- sucrose
- maltose
- dextrose
- fructose
- galactose
- high-fructose corn syrup
- agave nectar / syrup

- white sugar
- brown sugar
- cane sugar
- beet sugar
- barley malt
- caramel

Artificial sweeteners such as aspartame (also known under trade name NutraSweet®, Equal® and Equal-Measure®), saccharin and sucralose are even worse than sugar. They are known carcinogens; numerous studies into artificial sweeteners have found they destroy the gut microbiome, are linked to obesity, Type 2 diabetes and other metabolic dysfunctions. An in-depth review of the sweetener sucralose (Splenda®) published in the *Journal of Toxicology and Environmental Health* listed safety concerns such as DNA damage, toxicity and hormonal disruption when used in cooking (*Abou-Donia et al, 2008*).

Safer alternatives to sweeteners:

- raw honey
- stevia
- molasses
- date syrup

- coconut nectar
- coconut sugar
- coconut blossom

On the next page is an example of what the typical Briton has for breakfast — a cereal bar and juice.

### Kellogg's Special K Red Berry Bars, 27g

Shockingly, there are nine sugar ingredients in this one bar alone which is marketed as a 'protein' bar; it's not a protein bar at all based on that. If you feel you need a chemistry degree to understand the ingredients, put it down.

*Ingredients:* wholegrain oats (30%), sultanas and cranberries blend (23%; sultanas, sunflower oil), juice infused cranberries (cranberries, pineapple juice syrup, pineapple juice concentrate, sunflower oil), rice flour, glucose syrup, cereal crispies (7%) (wholewheat flour, rice flour, sugar, malted barley flour, malted wheat flour, salt, rapeseed oil, stabiliser (calcium carbonate), emulsifier (soy lecithin), wholewheat flakes (7%; whole wheat, sugar, salt, barley malt flavouring), sugar, corn fibre, maltodextrin, fructose, palm oil, humectant (glycerol), natural flavouring, strawberry juice concentrate, antioxidant (tocopherol rich extract), emulsifier (soy lecithin), skimmed milk powder, niacin, iron, vitamin B6, vitamin B2 (riboflavin), vitamin B1 (thiamin), folic acid, vitamin B12.

| Typical Values | Per 100g | Per bar, 27g |
|---|---|---|
| Carbohydrate | 73g | 20g |
| - of which sugars (look for this figure) | 28g | 7.6g |

To calculate the teaspoons of sugar, simply look at the amount of the sugar in question and divide by four to get the number of teaspoons per serving or per 100g.
28g divided 4 = 7 teaspoons per 100g
7.6 divided by 4 = 1.9 teaspoons sugar per bar.

**Tropicana® Orange Juice Smooth (300ml)** — a small, lunchtime-sized drink
*Ingredients:* 100% pure squeezed smooth orange juice.

| Typical Values | Per 100ml | Per 300ml |
|---|---|---|
| Carbohydrate | 8.9g | 26.7g |
| - of which sugars | 8.9g | 26.7g |

Calculating the amount of sugar: 26.7 divided by 4 = 6.7 teaspoons. That's a shocking amount of sugar in a small lunchtime sized juice drink when the National Health Service (NHS) recommends up to 30g sugar per day which is the equivalent of 7 and a half teaspoons for those aged 11 and over.[17]

Even though Tropicana® may argue that there is no added sugar and that it's filled with naturally occurring sugars, it still has the same

---

17 How much sugar is good for me? (2018) — www.nhs.uk/common-health-questions/ food-and-diet/how-much-sugar-is-good-for-me/

effect on blood sugar levels and the hormonal system. It elevates blood sugar levels much faster than the process of chewing and digesting food. Fruit juice is nothing but sugar water; the juice has long lost its nutritional value as it is no longer fresh. Opt for cold-pressed juices and ones that have a low fruit content and more vegetables.

Imagine you grab a small bottle of orange juice and a cereal 'protein' bar, and you've already consumed more than eight and a half teaspoons of sugar. It's therefore really important to know how to read labels at a glance as the food giants are very good at marketing their 'healthy' products to the public and children.

### Gluten

Gluten is the protein found in wheat, barley, spelt, rye and oats. Gluten intolerance or sensitivity arises when one cannot digest the protein portion of these gluten grains leading to an autoimmune response. Unfortunately, the medical industry tends to dismiss gluten intolerance unless you have coeliac disease. Coeliac disease is a digestive condition caused by an autoimmune reaction to gluten. The small intestine becomes inflamed and unable to absorb nutrients.[18] However, gluten sensitivity is one of the top intolerances that is diagnosed after food intolerance testing. Symptoms include bloating, gas, constipation, diarrhoea, headaches, fatigue and more.

*'We don't digest gluten completely, which is unlike any other protein. The immune system seems to see gluten as a component of bacteria and deploys weapons to attack it, and this creates some collateral damage we call inflammation.'* — Dr Alessio Fasano, Director of the Center for Coeliac Research and Treatment

Gluten can cause inflammation and inflammation is a precursor to most diseases. The undigested gluten proteins break down the microvilli (tiny, hair-like structures) that increase the surface area of the small intestine. This creates space between the villi, where food particles and pathogens can enter through the gut wall and into the bloodstream, leading to what is known as 'leaky gut syndrome'.

---

18 Overview Coeliac Disease (2016) — www.nhs.uk/conditions/coeliac-disease/

The food particles that enter the bloodstream create an autoimmune response, because they are seen as foreign by the body. The body then attacks itself — this is what autoimmunity is — thinking it's attacking these particles, adding more fuel to the fire of inflammation. The situation becomes chronic as the cycle continuously repeats itself whenever the gut is exposed to gluten.

For those suffering from any autoimmune disease such as hypothyroidism, lupus, arthritis, myalgic encephalitis (ME), chronic fatigue syndrome, fibromyalgia and joint pain, they should consider eliminating gluten from their diet altogether to allow time for the gut to heal. The immune system is located in the gut after all. I've seen vast improvements in clients with minor ailments to full-blown inflammatory diseases once they eliminate gluten from their diets. Something to note is that when gluten doesn't get digested properly, it turns into substances called gluteomorphins with a similar chemical structure to opiates — morphine and heroin — creating an addictive dependency on gluten foods. There has been a growing number of studies conducted by Reichelt *et al*, 1994 and Shattock *et al*, 1990, where gluteomorphins were detected in the urine of patients with schizophrenia, autism, ADHD, epilepsy, Down's syndrome, depression and autoimmune diseases like rheumatoid arthritis.

In any case, everyone can do with reducing their consumption of gluten. Having it now and again is something a healthy gut microbiome can deal with. Watch out for 'gluten-free' products; if the ingredient list is a bunch of chemical names you don't recognise, put it down. Foods made from gluten-free and ancient grains such as millet, amaranth, teff and buckwheat are better alternatives.

### Fish and Seafood

Avoid farmed fish. Fish farming methods are similar to those of commercial meat farming. The fish are fed grains, soy, antibiotics and other drugs, often in overcrowded conditions. Furthermore, nutritional data documents that half a fillet of farmed Atlantic salmon has five-and-a-half times more omega-6 fats than wild salmon, from their grain-based diet and food pellets, throwing the delicate ratio of omega 6:3 way out.[19] Ideal ratio of omega-6 to omega-3 is 1:1, yet it is more like 20:1 or even higher in the Western diet today (*Simpopoulos, 2016*). Omega-3 and -6 fats are essential fatty acids only obtained through the diet. Omega-3 fats are anti-inflammatory, whilst omega-6 are pro-inflammatory. Inflammation is essential for survival as it helps fight infection and protect against tissue damage. However, too much omega-6 can fuel inflammation. In the West, the consumption of omega-6 fats is already very high; it's found in vegetable oils such as sunflower oil, nuts, seeds, poultry, fish, meat and eggs. If you think you're increasing your essential omega-3 fats through eating farmed fish, you're wrong. Investigations into Norwegian salmon farms found layers of waste some 15 metres high full of bacteria, drugs and pesticides (*Mercola, 2016*). Jerome Ruzzin, a toxicology researcher confirms Norwegian environmentalist activist, Kurt Oddekalv who said that 'farmed salmon is one of the most toxic foods in the world'.[20] Avoid farmed salmon and fish at all costs and opt for wild-caught fish instead.

As the level of pollution rises in lakes, rivers and oceans you will have to be choosy as to which fish you eat. Sadly, most of the planet's waterways are now polluted and contaminated with toxic waste, heavy metals, agricultural and pharmaceutical waste and other chemicals that bio-accumulate in the tissues and flesh of all marine life. The higher up the food chain, the higher the accumulation. Although 15 years ago, fish was deemed a healthy food choice, I would only recommend sticking to wild / line-caught fish one to two times a week. Rotate which type of fish you eat to avoid accumulation of any one toxin and by all means, avoid farmed fish. The best choices are small, cold-water, fatty fish like anchovies, herring, sardines, mackerel and wild-caught Alaskan salmon. The worst, with the highest levels of mercury, are the big fish that eat other fish. Avoid shark, swordfish, king mackerel, Chilean seabass, canned albacore and yellowfin tuna. See chart on next page.

---

19 Self Nutrition Data; fish, salmon, Atlantic, farmed, raw nutrition facts and data (2018) — https://nutritiondata.self.com/facts/finfish-and-shellfish-products/4258/2
20 Leech, Joe. Wild vs Farmed Salmon: which type of salmon is healthier? (2018) — https://www.healthline.com/nutrition/wild-vs-farmed-salmon#fatty-acids

| Mercury Levels in Fish | | |
|---|---|---|
| **High** | **Medium** | **Low** |
| Crab (blue) | Bass (striped, black) | Arctic Cod |
| Grouper | Carp | Anchovies |
| Mackerel (King, | Cod (Alaskan) | Sardine — Scallop |
| Spanish, Gulf) | Croaker (white, | Catfish — Clam |
| Marlin | Pacific) | Crab (domestic) |
| Orange Roughy | Halibut (Pacific, | Crawfish / Crayfish |
| Salmon (Farmed, | Atlantic) | Croaker (Atlantic) |
| Atlantic) | Lobster | Flounder |
| Seabass (Chilean) | Mahi Mahi | Haddock (Atlantic) |
| Shark | Monkfish | Hake — Herring |
| Swordfish | Perch (freshwater) | Mackerel (N. Atlantic, |
| Tilefish | Sablefish | Chub) |
| Tuna (Ahi, yellowfin, | Skate | Whitefish |
| bigeye, blue, canned | Snapper | Perch |
| albacore) | Tuna (canned chunk | Plaice |
| | light, skipjack) | Pollock |
| | Sea Trout | Salmon (Canned, |
| | | fresh, wild) |
| | | Tilapia |
| | | Trout (Freshwater) |
| | | Shrimp |

\* Table taken from Natural Resources Defense Council (nrdc)21

On the next page is a chart I've created to simplify your optimal food choices. Stock up your kitchen pantry and fridge with foods from the regular column. As Paul Chek teaches us in Holistic Lifestyle Coaching, Level 2, you have three choices:[22]

1. Optimal choice
2. Suboptimal choice
3. Indifference

Optimal would be consuming foods mostly from the regular list. Suboptimal would be consuming mostly from the occasional list, and indifference would be to do nothing.

---

21 Natural Resources Defense Council — Mercury in Fish www.nrdc.org/sites/default/
  files/walletcard.pdf
22 The CHEK Institute — www.chekinstitute.com/chek-holistic-lifestyle-coach-program/

| | Avoid | Occasional (1 – 3 X Week) | Regular (Daily) |
|---|---|---|---|
| **Alcohol** | Beer, cocktails, liquor, dark spirits (rum), alcopops | Wine, clear spirits (gin, vodka, tequila) | |
| **Drinks** | Frappes, all fruit juices, fruit smoothies, tropical juices, fizzy drinks, store-bought hot chocolate / lattes etc., • non-organic coffee and tea, instant coffee | Organic coffee, tea, fruit teas, freshly juiced juices (keep low fruit content), homemade lattes | Herbal teas, freshly juiced vegetables, filtered water, coconut water, green juices, green supplement powders like spirulina, wheatgrass, chlorella, etc. |
| **Proteins** | Farmed fish, supermarket eggs, commercially farmed meat, processed meats such as salami, wafer-thin packet ham / chicken / turkey slices etc, pork pies, ◆ soya, processed whey protein powders, most protein bars | ♣ Pork — limit to one to two a week; shellfish, low-mercury fish, tinned fish; free-range eggs; wild Alaskan salmon, wild / line-caught fish | Organic poultry, lamb, beef, venison, game, organ meats; free-range organic eggs; organic bone broths |
| **Carbohydrates** | White potatoes, chips, fries, crisps, all breakfast cereals, cereal / diet bars, corn and soya, wheat, tropical fruit — grapes, pineapple, mango, dried fruits, raisins, pasta, couscous white rice, bagels, paninis croissants, sandwiches, cakes, pastries, crackers, processed cereals — rice cakes, Ryvita | Root vegetables — sweet potato, squash, beetroot, carrots, yams; black / wild rice; lentils, pulses; oatcakes, spelt, rye, sourdough bread and oats (if not gluten intolerant), ♣ mushrooms, peppers, aubergine, tomatoes Fruits — papaya, apples, pears, bananas, oranges, melon | Ancient grains — millet, buckwheat, quinoa, amaranth Vegetables — dark green leafy veg, kale, broccoli, spinach, chard, rocket, green beans, asparagus; cauliflower, fennel, pak choi, mustard greens, spring greens, cabbage, cucumbers, courgettes, celery, watercress, radish, nori wrap, sea vegetables, seaweed Fruits — avocados, grapefruit, lemons, limes, kiwi, organic berries |

| | Avoid | Occasional (1 – 3 X Week) | Regular (Daily) |
|---|---|---|---|
| **Fats and Oils** | Vegetable oils — safflower, sunflower, cottonseed, canola, rapeseed oil; peanuts, roasted / salted nuts; margarine, vegetable spreads, low-fat products; skimmed milk, semi-skimmed milk; trans fats, hydrogenated fats, deep fried foods, tempura | Cashews, pistachios, pasteurised full fat organic dairy | Coconut oil, organic ghee, organic virgin olive oil, duck fat, beef fat, organic full fat butter, olives, avocados, avocado oil, walnut oil, medium chain triglyceride (MCT) oil, macadamia nuts, pecans, walnuts, brazils, almonds, organic full fat dairy, raw milk, unpasteurised cheese, coconut milk, nut milks, nut butters, chia, hemp, pumpkin, sunflower seeds |
| **Sweets** | Sweets, confectionery, milk chocolate; any ingredient ending in -*ose* is a sugar: fructose, maltose, glucose, etc. | Dark chocolate (70 – 85%) cacao, Ω fat bombs | Dark chocolate (85% and above) |
| **Sauces** | Ketchup, BBQ sauce, most cooking sauces, soy, sweet chilli | | Tamari, coconut, hummus, homemade guacamole, olive tapenade |
| **Herbs** | Table salt (any bright white salt), pre-mixed herbs with ingredient listings you don't understand or with added salt | | Himalayan pink salt, unrefined sea salt, black pepper, coriander, parsley, thyme, rosemary, basil, mixed herbs, oregano, cardamom ginger, cayenne pepper, cinnamon, turmeric |

|  | Avoid | Occasional (1 – 3 X Week) | Regular (Daily) |
|---|---|---|---|
| **Superfoods/ Supplements** |  |  | Spirulina, chlorella, moringa, babao, acai, acerola, barley grass, wheatgrass, kamut, maca, lucuma, reishi, cordyceps mushrooms |
| **Fermented Foods** | Avoid fermented foods if you have bacterial/fungal/candida overgrowth in the gut |  | sauerkraut, kimchi, miso, tempeh, kefir, kombucha |

- Non-organic tea and coffee — conventional coffee is one of the most heavily sprayed foods in the world, closely followed by tea.

♦ Soya — one of the most genetically modified foods in the world and contains phytoestrogens that mimic oestrogen in the body. Choose only fermented soy products such as tofu, tempeh and miso.

♣ Pork — pigs do not have sweat glands and so naturally accumulate parasites. Avoid if your immune system is low.

♠ Mushrooms, aubergine, tomatoes, peppers, eggplant and paprika make up the nightshade family and can create an inflammatory reaction for anyone with an auto-immune disease or inflammation

Ω Fat bombs, see recipe on page 74

### *Food Rituals*

Give thanks for your food. Connect to it; it's nourishing you, your body, mind and soul. Eat slowly, chewing everything at least 15 times until liquid and then swallow. Avoid distractions. Put your phone away from your food to avoid electromagnetic stress and radiation. While your energy is focused on your phone, it's much harder to be in the parasympathetic state necessary for digestion. Make a clear space where you eat and put away any paperwork.

# Recipes

### *Brain smoothie*

*Serves one*

This is great to pack in your bag when you are on the go or even for breakfast. It contains lots of healthy fats to keep you satiated and improve cognitive function.

*Ingredients*

    ½ banana
    ½ avocado
    2 handfuls of blueberries
    handful walnuts (*optional*)
    handful of spinach
    250ml of almond / coconut / milk alternative

Simply blend for about 30 seconds until liquid and drink

### *Bone broth*

*Makes 3 – 4 litres (depending on size of cooker)*

Bone broth is incredibly healing for the gut lining and connective tissue, is easily digestible and is full of minerals and amino acids.

*Ingredients*

    2 – 3kgs chicken carcass / fish bones / beef bones / other animal bones
    filtered water
    1 tbsp apple cider vinegar
    *Optional —*
    pepper
    2 handfuls celery, sweet potato, onion, leeks, carrots
    a few dried bay leaves

*Directions*

1. Place the bones in a slow cooker. Pour in the filtered water to cover the bones

2. Add in the apple cider vinegar which helps to extract the minerals from the bones.

3. Peel and chop up vegetables and add to the broth with the bay leaves. Cover with lid.

4. Cook for at least eight to ten hours on low heat, six to eight hours on medium heat or five to six hours on high heat.

5. Strain the liquid using a sieve and enjoy. Once it cools, it will keep in the fridge for up to a week or freeze in glass containers to use during in the week.

### Fat bombs

Many protein balls, bars and snacks are made from dates, which drives up the sugar content, creating an insulin spike. If, like me, you have a sweet tooth, a fat bomb satisfies that and is great when energy levels are low. It's made from dense fats like coconut oil, cacao butter, nuts and seeds. Remember, fat is your friend. It's best eaten on its own and not with sugar. I've selected my two favourite, easy-to-make recipes below.

### Chocolate fat bomb truffles

Recipe from Jennafer Ashley of PaleoHacks.[23]

*Cooking time: ten minutes*

*Servings: approximately 12*

*Ingredients*

　　1 tbsp vanilla extract

　　2 small ripe avocados

　　120g raw cacao powder

　　2 tbsp raw cacao powder for dusting

　　3 tbsp coconut oil, melted

　　1½ tbsp raw honey, maple or date syrup

*Directions*

1. In a mixing bowl, combine the melted coconut oil, avocado, vanilla and honey. Use a hand mixer on medium speed to mix the ingredients until they reach a smooth consistency.

---

23 Tasty chocolate and avocado truffles recipe (2017) — https://recipes.mercola.com/avocado-truffles-recipe.aspx

2. Gradually mix in 120g of the raw cacao powder until it completely combines with the other ingredients. Place in the freezer for ten minutes.

3. Using a tablespoon, scoop out the mixture and roll it into balls. Dust with the 2 tbsp of cacao powder.

4. Store in the refrigerator, then serve once chilled.

### Coconut, lime and mint ball

This is a favourite of mine from Jasmine Hemsley.[24]

*Ingredients*

> 200g ground almonds
> 140g desiccated coconut
> 2 tbsp maple syrup
> zest of 2 unwaxed limes
> ½ tsp vanilla extract
> 1 tsp peppermint extract / oil
> 100g coconut oil
> pinch of salt

*Directions*

1. Blitz the almonds, 60g of the desiccated coconut, maple syrup, zest, vanilla extract, peppermint extract, coconut oil and sea salt in a food processor / nutribullet until chunky but evenly mixed.

2. Taste the mixture and add a drop or more of the peppermint extract if needed, then blitz again.

3. Take small pieces from the bowl and roll them into 12 – 15 balls with the palms of your hands. Refrigerate for around 20 minutes, until firm.

4. Spread out the remaining desiccated coconut and roll each ball in it until completely covered. Store somewhere cool or in the fridge for up to a week.

---

24 Hemsley, J (2017) East by West, Bluebird, London

### Health Bank Deposits

✓ Prioritise all animal products to adhere to organic / biodynamic practices

✓ Make all on the dirty dozen list organic

✓ Make your own veggie wash and wash your fruit and veg

✓ Consume wild / line-caught, low-mercury fish

✓ Look up your local farmers' market(s) and organic food delivery / farm boxes

✓ Consume most of your food from the regular / daily column in the food chart earlier in this section

✓ Eat full fat instead of skimmed / semi-skimmed / low-fat produce

✓ Avoid all refined grains and processed sugars such as white flour, cereals, cakes, pastries, biscuits, confectionery, crackers

✓ Get familiar with reading labels and knowing the sugar content in so-called healthy snacks

✓ Apply the 80 / 20 rule. Eat most of your foods from the daily list 80% of the time and the rest 20% of the time.

✓ Eat in a calm and quiet environment to stimulate the parasympathetic pathway required for digestion

✓ Drink a glass of water with juice squeezed from a quarter of a lemon 15 minutes before your meal to aid digestion

✓ Make your own bone broth and freeze into batches for the week

✓ Rotate your foods every four days to avoid food intolerances

✓ Give thanks for your food before every meal.

# Water

The human body is made up of approximately 70% water. Throughout the day, water is lost through breathing, urination and sweating. It's important to replenish with adequate amounts of *quality* water every day as dehydration has a significant impact on cellular function, health and cognition. To work out your daily water intake, use this equation:

Bodyweight (kgs) x 0.033 = litres of water / day
For example, a 70kg woman (70kgs x 0.033) requires 2.3 litres / day

*'Water's chief function is to maintain a stable environment inside*
*and outside the cells, acquiring sufficient nutrition*
*and aiding elimination of waste in cells.'* — Paul Chek

An article published by Brunel University in 2016, reported that a significant amount of medicines were excreted into water.[25] John Sumpter, Professor of Ecotoxicology at Brunel University, made this statement about strong psycho-active drugs like antidepressants in the environment:

*'Once they get into the water system,*
*they retain their powerful biological activity'.*

It has long been documented that the altered sex and reproductive characteristics in fish and other marine creatures is as a result of waste chemicals and higher levels of oestrogen in the water supply. Although concerns have been raised, the truth is no one knows what the long-term effects of a lifelong intake of drugs at low concentrations are. I know that I do not want to put myself or my future children forward to be human guinea pigs.

A study carried out by a team at King's College, London in 2019 revealed high concentrations of cocaine polluting the River Thames due to the high use of the drug in London.[26] Londoners are amongst the highest users of cocaine in any city. A separate study published by

25 Brunel University London; Is Tap water safe to drink? (2016) — www.brunel.ac.uk/ research/News-and-events/news/Is-tap-water-safe-to-drink
26 Independent; Record cocaine levels in Thames probably not making fish high, experts say (2019) — www.independent.co.uk/news/uk/home-news/cocaine-london-river-thames-water-research-kings-college-study-fish-high-drugs-a8738146.html

the University of Naples Federico II found eels to become hyperactive and breakdown musculoskeletal tissue when exposed to small doses of cocaine in the water (*Capaldo et al, 2018*). Cocaine and other drugs are therefore making their way into the drinking water supply through human excretion and roughly 80,000 lines of coke are ending up in the River Thames every day, with the highest amount during the week. Everything else aside, what does that say about modern-day stress and working culture?

*'Water utilities are failing to remove cocaine from waste water, which means our water courses are likely to see ever increasing levels of drug residue. If cocaine isn't effectively removed, we can be sure that other drug residues will also be getting through.'* — Roger Wiltshire, MD of Pure H2O[27]

Human behaviour has polluted almost every single water supply in the world with chemicals from commercial farming, non-biodegradable household products, cosmetics, pharmaceutical and recreational drugs that cannot be broken down. Half of all women and men in England are on prescription medication, with a significant proportion on at least three different types, the most common being antidepressants, statins and painkillers. How can water treatment plants possibly keep up with this level of pollutants and contaminants? Instead, chemicals chlorine and fluoride are added, and that ends up in our bodies.

### Solutions

1. The best water in the world is from a natural spring. It is filtered through the earth containing nature's minerals. Go to www.findaspring.com for your nearest spring, take some big glass bottles / jugs and fill up. There are a few in and around London.

2. Invest in a Berkey® filter to filter your drinking water. It filters 99.99 per cent of chlorine, viruses, harmful pathogenic bacteria, drug residues, heavy metals, parasites and other impurities while leaving behind the essential minerals your body needs. This is unlike other filter techniques such as reverse osmosis,

---

27 Cocaine in River Thames highlights water pollution concerns (2019) — www.pureh2o.co.uk/cocaineriverthames/

which strips the water of all minerals. You can also separately get fluoride filters through Berkey, to filter fluoride added to the water supply, which is known as a neurotoxin.

3.  Buy bottled water in glass where you can that comes from artesian wells or springs. Plastic leaches into water.

4.  Have your own refillable stainless steel / glass / BPA free bottle that you can fill up from your Berkey filter.

5.  Add a pinch of Himalayan / sea salt to each litre of water to add minerals.

6.  If you are out and about filling up from a tap, add a charcoal filter stick to your drinking bottle; it's very effective at removing chlorine, heavy metals and other organic compounds leaving the minerals behind. However, it will not filter all pathogens or pharmaceutical drug residues.

7.  Make your own filter very cheaply by filling up a jug of water, adding shungite crystals and a charcoal stick and leave for two to three hours. Shungite has the ability to clean water of most compounds and even radioactive elements, according to researchers at Rice University and the Kazan Federal University in Russia.[28]

### Health Bank Deposits

✓  Work out how much water you need to drink per day using the formula provided in this section.

✓  Go to www.findaspring.com for a spring near you

✓  Invest in a home water filter like a Berkey®

✓  Add a pinch of Himalayan / sea salt to add minerals back into the water

✓  Use a charcoal stick and shungite crystals to filter water

✓  Carry a refillable glass / stainless steel or BPA-free, refillable water bottle

✓  Opt for eco-friendly and biodegradable cleaning products and cosmetics that do not pollute the waters (see Detoxify Your Home)

✓  Bonus — invest in a water filtration system for your entire home

---

28 Rice University 'Treated carbon pulls radioactive elements from water: Researchers have developed unique sorbents, target Fukushima accident site' (2017) — www.sciencedaily.com/releases/2017/01/170119134534.htm

## Movement — Working In vs Working Out

The first time I came across the concept of 'working in' was through Paul Chek's teachings in *How to Eat, Move and Be Healthy (2014)*. In a society so obsessed with 'doing, doing, doing', there is little room to 'just be'. It's become almost a badge of honour as to who had the least amount of sleep last night and the most duties to fulfil! Our nervous systems are so overwhelmed with digital stimulation, endless lists of things to do, achieving and looking good all at the same time. Most of the clients that I coach in London are very stressed, work hard, lead demanding lifestyles, lack energy and are pretty burnt out. When clients come to me with a high-stress profile (which most of them do), the last thing they need is to work *out* hard. They need to work *in* and cultivate their life force. There are many, many books about working out and different training methods, hence why I am going to focus only on 'working in'.

Movement is one of the six foundational pillars of health. Like animals, we need to move our bodies every day, to help move stagnant energy and facilitate the pumping systems of the body. Activities such as Tai Chi, Qigong, restorative and yin yoga, breathwork and mobilisation exercises all help to draw in energy, sending vitality to the organs and replenishing your batteries.

*'Aging can be seen ultimately as a decline in the life force or vitality, with death at the end point of this decline. Thus, cultivating your life force and vitality is one of the most valuable resources in turning back the biological clock.'* — Master Fong Ha,
famous expert of Tai Chi and Qigong

In Paul Chek's *How to Eat, Move and Be Healthy*, he states that 'the slower you move your body, the faster your chi energy / life force moves delivering beneficial energy to the hormonal, organ and glandular systems. The faster you move the slower the chi energy / life force moves.' Working in also helps to balance the right and left brain hemispheres.

When you work out, you are expending energy and thus need to have enough energy reserves to replenish, repair and reap the benefits from your training. The benefits of training happen while you rest. Think about when you do an intense training session, you wake up with muscle soreness. While you sleep your tissues and muscles are repairing. Training on an empty tank will result in you feeling more exhausted and fatigued because there are not enough reserves to replenish and reap the goodness from your training. Thus, focusing on forms of exercise or activities that 'draw' energy in and cultivate your life force, topping up your fuel tank, is vital. Working out is not bad but with a population in the city suffering from fatigue and burnout, you cannot do everything at a high intensity. There needs to be the *yin* and the *yang*; *yang* is the doing, the action, and the *yin* is the being, restoration, nourishment and healing. Those living in cities are predominantly too *yang*, and too much *yang* will result in disease and illness.

A typical example is the city guy: he works hard, long hours and has to entertain clients out until late with dinner and drinks. He socialises hard to let off steam, drinking large amounts of alcohol. When he trains, he smashes it hard in the gym, probably training for an ultra-marathon or some kind or triathlon. Then he has a heart attack or, worse still, drops dead out of the blue in his late 30s or early 40s and everyone wonders why because he was 'so fit'. This is why we really need to evaluate our definition of health; is it based on outward appearance, or harmony of body, mind and spirit? The body cannot handle this much physiological load; it will eventually shut down and that will manifest itself as an illness of some sort. You cannot keep draining the batteries without recharging them, hence the need to regularly work in.

The year 2016 was particularly challenging for me. I'd saved enough money to put a deposit on a flat. Although very exciting and a great position to be in, I was full of fear. The property prices in London are incredibly high and the opportunity to buy somewhere in my budget was very scarce, with fierce competition. Would I be able to afford to stay in London and how would I serve my one-to-one clients and keep my business going if not? Would I have to start all over again in a completely new area, this time with the pressure of a mortgage? I moved three times in one year while I was flat hunting, not knowing where I was going next or how long I would need to stay. I was in romantic relationships that were going nowhere. I had no stability in any area of my life and felt completely ungrounded, stuck and full of fear and anxiety. While all my friends were settling down, getting married, buying houses with their respective partners and having children, I was 34, single, dating non-committal men, running my own business, trying to do everything on my own and tired of always being the 'strong one' and holding it all together. Every time I went to a social event or gathering, friends and parents of friends would ask, 'When are you going to settle down?' 'When are you going to have a baby?' It was so inappropriately far from where I was; I would brush it off but, inside, I felt very low and left behind.

At the same time, I had a full practice of one-to-one personal training and bodywork clients. I was giving out so much energy and trying to hold it all together at a time when I needed to step back and take time for myself. I continued to do my own training in the gym, but my body was giving me some warning signs. I kept feeling twinges in my back and so I would back off. This was very unusual for me as I rarely had injuries. I knew immediately it was linked to my emotional state of mind. I would leave it a day or two and then go back to doing some training. I participated in an obstacle race event and, after doing some tyre flips, I felt my back 'go'. It didn't feel right but I continued the event anyway and completed it. The stubborn part of me and the part that wanted to push, strive and achieve didn't want to give in, even though I knew all I knew; I felt like I'd be letting myself down.

*Big Mistake.* The next day I was in absolute agony; it felt as if I had a knife stabbing me in the centre of my lower back. I could barely lift myself out of bed and it was painful to go to the toilet. I had sacroiliac joint dysfunction (the major joint in the body that holds the lower back and pelvis in place), which can cause sciatica. I had agonising episodes over the next 18 months. Still, to this day, it's not quite the same, but so much better now and it's a long time since I've had any agonising episodes, thanks to my partner Warren who is a master at injury rehabilitation. This was my biggest lesson; when the body talks, you *must* listen. I know so much better now and this was a time when I should have definitely been only working in. The wisdom of the body will manifest an injury, illness or disease as a way of making you slow down.

Later that year, on my CHEK Holistic Lifestyle Level 2 Coaching Training, I learnt that the lower back is linked to the adrenal glands (where we hold fear). It is also linked to stability, security, being grounded, rooted and supported — all of the things that were up in the air for me. It's no surprise I had manifested this injury. The best thing I could have done during this period was to work in more to cultivate my life force and help me increase my resilience to stress. Needless to say, I learnt my lesson and am very good now at taking a step back when I need self-care time and working in.

I recommend my clients work in on the days their energy levels feel pretty low. A work in programme or activity is great to do in the evening to help bring the body into a more parasympathetic state and unwind from the day, or even in the morning to help feel grounded and centred for the day ahead. Slow diaphragmatic breathing as suggested on page 30 is a wonderful way to bring more energy / chi / life force in.

On the next few pages are examples of a work in programme that can be done anywhere. Breathe in and out through the nose to induce more of a parasympathetic state, with the eyes closed if you can. The movements are done slowly.

## *Example one*

| Exercise | Reps | Tempo |
|---|---|---|
| Neck rotations (*pic. 1, 2*) | up to 20 each direction | slow, breathing pace |
| Shoulder rotations (*pic. 3, 4, 5*) | 10 each direction | breathing pace, inhale as arms go back and exhale as arms come forward |
| Egyptian arms (*pic. 6, 7*) | 10 each side | breathing pace |
| Spinal mobilisations (*pic. 8, 9*) | 5 each direction | exhale as you sit back on your heels, inhale as you come forwards toward the wrists |
| Low lunge and side twist (*pic. 10, 11*) | 5 each side | breathing pace |
| T-stretch (*pic. 12, 13*) | 10 each side | breathing pace, exhale as leg comes across body, inhale as it lifts away |

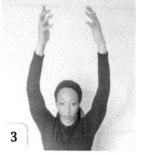

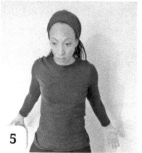

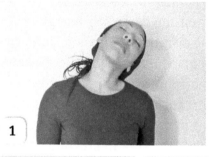

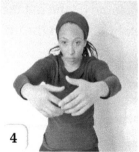

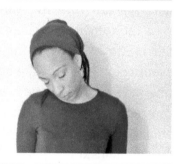

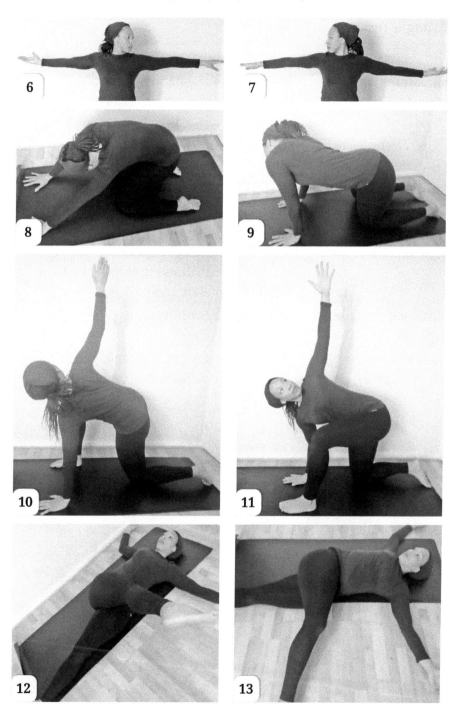

## Example two

| Exercise | Reps | Tempo |
|---|---|---|
| Breathing squat (*pic. 14, 15*) | 10 – 30 | 4 seconds down / pause / 4 seconds up. Exhale as you lower, inhale as you come up |
| Alternating leg drop (*pic. 16, 17*) | 10 each side | slow |
| Kneeling camel opener (*pic. 18, 19, 20, 21*) | 10 each side | breathing pace, inhale as arm sweeps up, exhale down |
| Cat cow (*pic. 22, 23*) | 6 of each | breathing pace, inhale arching through the spine. exhale to cat, drawing chin to chest and pelvis under |
| Thoracic mobilisations (*pic. 24, 25*) | 10 each direction | breathing pace |
| Jaw release (*pic. 26, 27, 28*) | 3 | slow yawn applying pressure downwards on either side of the jaw |

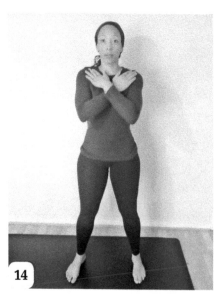

14

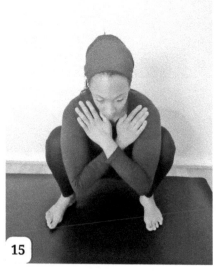

15

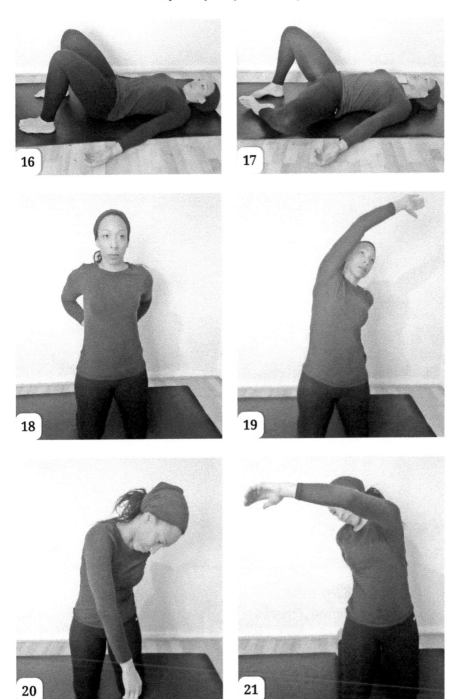

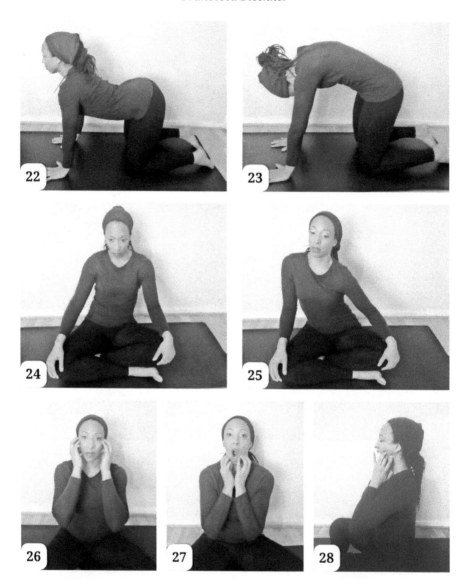

### Health Bank Deposits

✓ Research to see if there are any Tai chi, Qigong, restorative / yin / slow flow yoga classes near you

✓ Take a ten-minute break in the day and implement the work in programme into your day between tasks. Begin to tune into your body as to how often you need to do it

# Detoxify Your Home

Physiological stress is not just as a result of emotional factors, but also because of the stress the liver is under to detoxify and break down toxic chemical ingredients. Many of these are inhaled, such as formaldehyde, synthetic fragrances, triclosan and other volatile organic compounds (VOCs). VOCs are compounds that easily become vapours or gases, such as fumes from paint.

A recent study by the environment charity Global Action Plan (GAP) in 2019 found indoor air pollution to be 3.5 times worse than that outside in the UK and described UK homes as 'indoor pollution boxes'.[29] Pollution particles from outdoor transport, burning stoves and open-wood fires are also contributing factors.

The tiny particles can be harmful to health as they can enter the bloodstream and vital organs. As mentioned earlier, toxins are stored in fat and the more toxins that accumulate in your body, the more fat you will hold onto to protect against these toxins getting to your vital organs. Chemical toxic compounds wreak havoc on the hormonal system and are major contributing factors to adrenal fatigue, chronic fatigue, fibromyalgia, asthma, brain fog and weight gain — to name a few. We may not be able to control outdoor pollution, but there are certainly many things we can take action on to improve our indoor air pollution and exposure to chemical toxins. Animals and children breathe much faster than adults and have smaller bodies, so the impact of inhaling and ingesting chemicals is likely more significant and potentially harmful (*Strauss, 2016*). It is our duty to clean up the household environment, especially if you have a young family.

In the next section, **Space Clearing**, you will see which plants are best to have for mopping up indoor air pollution. Diffusing essential oils and Himalayan salt lamps also help. On the next page is a list of chemicals found in household ingredients and their side effects.

---

29 UK homes 'toxic boxes' due to indoor air pollution (2019) — www.airqualitynews. com/2019/05/15/uk-homes-toxic-boxes-due-to-indoor-air-pollution/

## *Chemicals in Household Cleaning Products*

| Chemical Ingredient / Product | Found in | Potential Risks / Effects | Natural Alternative |
|---|---|---|---|
| Chlorine | Multi-purpose cleaners, liquid bleaches, washing powders / detergents | Irritates eyes and lungs, can trigger asthma attacks, aggravates respiratory system; 1990 Clean Air Act lists chlorine as a hazardous air pollutant | Make your own multi-purpose cleaner; biodegradable washing powders and detergents |
| Fragrances | These are petrochemicals found in air fresheners, scented candles, laundry / washing detergents | Itchy eyes, skin irritation, headaches, wheezing, asthma, chronic chemical sensitivity, lethargy, short-term memory loss | Diffuse essential oils instead of air fresheners / plug-ins; use soy / beeswax candles infused with essential oils; choose un-fragranced products; mix lavender essential oil or rose with water in spray bottle and spray clothes before washing |
| VOCs | Liquid cleaners, household products, paints, glass cleaners, artificial fragrances, plug-ins and spray air fresheners (VOCs are the strong scents that come from products) | Intoxication, drowsiness, breathing difficulties, asthma attacks, skin and eye irritation, disorientation and headaches; long-term exposure can damage the nervous system | Low-VOC paints, diffuse organic essential oils; make your own multi-purpose spray |

| Chemical Ingredient / Product | Found in | Potential Risks / Effects | Natural Alternative |
|---|---|---|---|
| Triclosan | Anti-bacterial and anti-fungal household products | Hormonal disruptor affecting oestrogen and thyroid; contributes to the development of resistant superbugs | Spray bottle with water and tea tree oil, lemons to clean chopping boards, etc. |
| Bleach and ammonia | Bleach, toilet cleaner | Produces toxic fumes, highly toxic to eyes, nose, throat, lungs and skin, asthma, respiratory issues | Make your own toilet cleaner |

### Making Your Own Natural Household Products

It's so easy to make your own products; you'll need only a few staple ingredients some of which will be multi-purpose, saving you money and contributing to a cleaner environment. Make sure you are not using old household cleaning containers to avoid a chemical contamination / crossover that can be toxic.

### Multi-purpose cleaner

Use for spraying kitchen and bathroom countertops, kitchen stoves, cabinets, dining tables and chairs.

*What you need:*
    500ml spray bottle
    2 tbsp liquid Castile soap
    5 – 10 drops tea tree / lemon / thieves essential oil
    500ml water

*Directions:*
    Add the liquid Castile soap and essential oils in the spray bottle then add the water and shake well.

## Toilet cleaner[30]

*What you need:*

    60ml liquid Castile soap

    5 drops of peppermint and lemon essential oil

    1tbsp white vinegar

    30mls water in a squirty bottle

*Directions:*

    Place soap and essential oils into squirty bottle with 30mls water and shake well. Add the white vinegar, mixing well. Squeeze mixture into the toilet bowl and leave to work for an hour. Scrub with toilet brush and flush.

## Laundry powder

*What you need:*

    250ml washing soda (usually in the laundry aisle at the bottom)

    250ml borax

    1 bar of natural soap (I like Dr Bronner's® scented with essential oils)

    *Optional* 5 – 10 drops essential oil lemon / lavender / rose

*Directions:*

    Take a bar of natural soap and grate it with a cheese grater or chop it into chunks and put it into a food processor. If putting it in a food processor, wait a minute or two before removing the top so as to not inhale the dust from the soap. Add the grated soap to the washing soda and borax. Mix well. Place in an airtight container and use 1 – 2 tbsp per load.

    Baking soda is also a great stable to have for cleaning worktops, bathtubs and grime off stoves etc. Simply sprinkle a little onto a damp cloth and use to gently scrub grease, grime, food spills and water marks. Rinse well with warm water to avoid a powdery residue. Coconut oil is also great as a wood polisher and lubricant for doors. There are many resources on how to make your own natural household products or look for eco-friendly household cleaning products to buy. Above are just a few of the most commonly used.

---

30 Strauss, R (2016) The Natural Household Cleaner, IMM Lifestyle Books, UK

## Cookware and microwaves

There is a lot of cookware out there that is toxic and it's good to know what to look out for. Non-stick and Teflon®-coated pans, pots and bakeware have a synthetic coating of polytetrafluoroethylene (PTFE). When heated the chemical called perfluorooctanoic acid (PFOA) is released. PFOA is toxic to the body and has been linked to an array of health conditions including kidney and testicular cancer (Barry *et al*, 2013) and thyroid, liver disease and decreased fertility.[31]

In a public health statement by The Agency for Toxic Substances & Disease Registry (ATSDR), it was stated that,

*"Once in your body, perfluoroalkyls tend to remain unchanged for long periods of time. The most commonly used perfluoroalkyls (PFOA and PFOS) stay in the body for many years".*[32]

The company Chemours (formerly known as DuPont) owns the Teflon brand. They knowingly kept documented evidence of the health risks to humans and the environment for decades from the public,[33] and contaminated the world's drinking water supply with perfluorinated chemicals. The company was fined $16.5 million by the US Environmental Protection Agency in 2005. PFOA is no longer used in the manufacturing process of Teflon products. As we are coming to an age of sustainability and conscious consumerism, it is worth questioning the ethics behind the company and the products they are making now, even if they are PFOA-free? I highly recommend watching the documentary *The Devil We Know* about the DuPont cover up.

You will notice that the coating on some cheap pans begins to flake after some use. If cooking at a high heat, the chemicals in the coating may then leach into your food when you are cooking and end up in your body. Dispose and replace old, flaking and scratched pans. In addition, avoid aluminium, copper and ceramic-coated cookware and

---

31 US Department of Health and Human Services: Tox guide for perfluoroalkyls (2018) — www.atsdr.cdc.gov/toxguides/toxguide-200.pdf
32 Public Health Statement, Perfluoroalkyls (August, 2015) — www.atsdr.cdc.gov/toxprofiles/tp200-c1-b.pdf
33 United States Environmental Protection Agency: E.I. DuPont de Nemours and Company PFOA Settlements — www.epa.gov/enforcement/ei-dupont-de-nemours-and-company-pfoa-settlements

cooking in aluminium foil. Aluminium is linked to some neurological disorders including Alzheimer's. Even if these pans are coated, the coating does not last forever and often chips, exposing the heavy metals underneath that can leach into your food. Many ceramic coated pans have aluminium underneath. Even though many non-stick cookware brands are going PFOA and PTFE free, they may be using other perfluoroalkyl and polyfluoroalkyl substances (PFAs). The research on this is conflicting and it's best to avoid non-stick cookware altogether as there are better options out there. The best cookware items are cast iron pans, enamel coated cast iron, stainless steel (look for the numbers 18 / 0, 18 / 8 or 18 / 10 at the bottom), glass and 100% ceramic cookware, *not* ceramic coated.

Avoid microwaves; the cell wall of foods become so damaged by the waves produced by these ovens that the gut receptors barely recognise microwaved food particles, causing an immune reaction (*David Getoff, 2001*).

### Cosmetics and make-up

In a study published by Bionsen, a natural deodorant company, it was found that the average woman puts 515 chemicals on her body every day.[34] Make-up, perfumes, lotions, mascara and other beauty products make up a toxic cocktail of thickeners, emulsifiers, colours and fragrances. With skin being the largest organ of the body, these chemicals and heavy metals are being absorbed straight into the bloodstream. Many of these ingredients cause hormonal disruption, immune dysfunction and are known carcinogens.

Fortunately, in the past decade, consumers have become more conscious of ingredients in beauty products and cosmetics and are opting for more natural and organic products. There are many natural and chemical-free skincare and body care products on the market to choose from. However, many of the bigger brands have jumped on the bandwagon, promising 'natural' and organic ingredients. This means very little in an industry that is loosely regulated.

---

34 Rice, M Revelaed... the 515 chemicals women put on their bodies every day (2009) — www.dailymail.co.uk/femail/beauty/article-1229275/Revealed--515-chemicals-women-bodies-day.html

Here is a breakdown of just some of the common chemicals found in cosmetics to avoid. For more detailed listings, please check out my recommended resources at the end of this book.

| Chemical Ingredient | Found In | Potential Risks / Effects | Natural Alternative |
|---|---|---|---|
| Formalde-hyde | Nail polish, soap, shampoo, hair growth preparations, keratin hair treatments. Used to preserve dead bodies! | Carcinogenic, fibromyalgia, fatigue, neurological damage | Organic, chemical-free products |
| Phthalates | Perfumes, deodorants, nail polish, hair mousses, gels and sprays | Linked to breast cancer; can harm reproductive organs; damage to the liver, kidney and lungs | Essential oils, Castile soap, coconut oil, shea butter, cocoa butter |
| Parabens (Methyl, Propyl / Butyl / Ethyl) | Many beauty and cosmetic products | Hormonal disruptor linked to breast cancer; can cause irritation and allergic reaction | Paraben-free products, Castile soap |
| Synthetic fragrances | Perfumes, colognes, soaps, hair sprays and other scented products | Hormonal disruptors; many are petroleum-based and can cause cancer, birth defects, central nervous system and behavioural disorders and allergic reactions | Essential oils, unfragranced products |
| Sodium lauryl / Laureth Sulfate (SLS) | Shampoos, body washes, bubble baths, toothpastes; creates the lathering effect | Skin and eye irritant; damages skin barrier function; enhances allergic response to other allergens and toxins; alters skin cells | Castile soap, Dead Sea / Epsom / Himalayan salts, SLS-free products, coconut oil for toothpaste, natural toothpaste |

| Chemical Ingredient | Found In | Potential Risks / Effects | Natural Alternative |
|---|---|---|---|
| Aluminium | Deodorants, anti-perspirants, loose powder | Highly toxic to the brain; linked to breast cancer | Deodorant paste / stick / stone; use anti-bacterial essential oils like lavender / tea tree or make your own with baking soda, arrowroot powder, coconut oil and essential oils |
| Fluoride | Toothpaste | US EPA National Health and Environmental Effects Research Laboratory have classified fluoride as a 'chemical having substantial evidence of developmental neurotoxicity'[35] | Fluoride-free toothpaste or make your own by mixing coconut oil, baking soda, pinch of Himalayan salt and peppermint essential oils |
| Chlorine, bleach, dioxin, pesticides, glues and dyes | Tampons and sanitary wear | Dioxin associated with suppressed immune system, tumours in abdomen and reproductive organs; hormone disruptor | Organic cotton tampons — brands Natracare®, Dame® |

By switching out some of the more commercial products to more natural alternatives where you can (or even making your own), you will radically reduce your chemical consumption. You'll also find you'll minimise your cosmetic product stack, as many natural alternatives double up as a few things. I stopped wearing perfume more than ten years ago. I became short of breath and wheezy when I did. Now, I stick to pure essentials oils as my perfume and people always ask me what fragrance I'm wearing. There is also a great app called Giki® that you can download to your phone and scan products when you go shopping. It will tell you how sustainable and ethical a product is.

---

35 Chocolate better for your teeth than fluoride (2013) — https://articles.mercola.com/sites/articles/archive/2013/11/19/chocolate-vs-fluoride-toothpaste.aspx

## Clothing

Natural and sustainable products like bamboo, cotton, hemp, merinho, linen and silk are a great option. A lot of clothing, especially sportswear, is made from synthetic, non-breathable materials like polyester and nylon which are really just plastics. Plastics, of course, contain xenoestrogens that mimic oestrogen in the body. Not all my clothing is made from natural materials, I just do my best where I can but prioritise my bedsheets, nightwear and underwear to be made of natural materials, as these are closest to my skin.

### Health Bank Deposits

✓ Invest in cast iron, stainless steel (look for 18/0, 18/8 or 18/10 at the bottom) or ceramic pans; never non-stick. The best is Saladmaster® — pricey but lasts a lifetime

✓ Dispose of old, chipped and flaking non stick cookware and pans

✓ Avoid microwaves

✓ Never use plastic spoons or utensils when cooking hot food. Opt for wooden, bamboo or stainless steel

✓ Make your own cleaning products with essential oils and natural ingredients or buy eco-friendly household cleaning products

✓ Use essential oils for perfume

✓ Choose fluoride-free toothpaste or make your own

✓ Make your own deodorant or buy a deodorant paste. Avoid sprays and aluminium-containing deodorants.

✓ Source cosmetics with all-natural organic ingredients; remember skin is the largest organ in the body. What you put on your skin is absorbed into your bloodstream

✓ Download the Giki® app and scan items while you shop

✓ Look for low VOC paint when decorating.

# Space Clearing

A clear space = a clear mind.

Ever since I was a young child, I would have the urge to declutter — must be the Virgo in me. My mum kept *everything*, and I would feel the need to clear out old magazines, bathroom products, the pantry, old books no longer read and clothes no longer worn. I just wanted to create a clearer space and mind and feel more expansive — a true minimalist.

Having moved so many times in London, and at one time having most of my belongings in storage when buying my flat, I became the queen of decluttering, getting rid of 'stuff' along the way. It's amazing that when most of my stuff was in storage and I was living temporarily in places, I actually really needed very little. Every time I moved, I gave clothes and shoes away that I hadn't worn for years, gave away things in storage that I hadn't missed and books that could be passed on. I went through boxes of photos (from the days we used to print photos) and threw away those that were of random people I didn't know, or blurry pictures, and kept the ones that held dear memories.

When I moved into my own flat, it was so easy to unpack and settle in; I had everything I needed with space and openness for energy to flow (key principle of feng shui). Now, when people come to my home, the first thing they say is, 'it has a great energy here'. Being grounded and centred is key for me, and the work I do with my clients. Having a clear, uncluttered space helps me to focus, stay clear, centred, expansive and relaxed.

I really enjoy decluttering and tidying up as I find it really satisfying. After my sister split with her partner, she asked me to help her declutter and clear her flat. We bagged up books and clothes for charity, gave boxes of old CDs away to a neighbour and reorganised her bookshelf to make it clearer. We took broken items to the tip and items for recycling, burned sage and palo santo, two powerful spiritual clearing and cleansing scents to clear and uplift the energy of her home. Instantly her space was transformed, feeling more spacious, expansive and peaceful.

## Clear the Air

Plants and foliage are a great way to brighten the home, especially if green space is limited in the city. Many city dwellers do not have a garden or very limited garden space; adding some green into your home has very healing benefits. Green is the colour for healing which is why nature is green. Plants release oxygen, helping to purify the air, even more important if you live near a main road. Open windows to circulate fresh air and if you do live by a busy main road, have lots of green plants nearby. According to NASA, indoor air is more polluted than outdoor air from airborne toxins, dust, germs, household chemicals and off-gassing from materials and appliances. Plants are very effective at cleaning indoor air and absorbing toxins. I love to have fresh flowers and plants in the home. The best green plants known to be excellent air purifiers are:[36]

- Spider
- Dracaenas
- Golden pathos
- Chrysanthemums
- Bamboo
- English ivy
- Boston Fern

## Scents, Oils, Diffusers

Everything is energy and everything has a vibration/frequency. You can raise the vibrational frequency of your home by using scents and diffusing essential oils in an air purifier. My personal favourites for the home are frankincense, sandalwood, geranium, patchouli, lemongrass (very refreshing) and lavender. Peppermint is great for studying and to awaken your senses. Both peppermint and lemon are great for cleaning the air. Not only do essential oils purify the air, they have beneficial effects on mood and stress levels. I do love a beautiful scented candle made with organic essential oils. Watch out for synthetically fragranced and paraffin wax candles (the majority on the market). Paraffin candles

---

36 The best air-purifying plants for your home (2016) — www.healthline.com/health/air-purifying-plants

are a petroleum by-product that burns a toxic, carcinogenic flame (definitely not good for those with respiratory issues). Beeswax and soy candles are the best with no synthetic fragrances, only essential oils.

I love to burn incense too; look for hand-rolled incense that doesn't contain any synthetic fragrances. Most of them do and they give me a headache when I burn them. I love The Henna Den's incense which are beautiful, natural hand-rolled incense sticks that waft a wonderful warming scent in the home.[37] My favourites are the big cleanse, wood spice, white sage, frankincense and oudh. First thing in the morning I will burn incense or diffuse essential oils to infuse through my home. Check out my recommended resources at the back for some of my favourite places to buy essential oils, incense and scents.

### Spiritual Cleansing Scents

In ancient Native American traditions, the herb sage is used in ceremonies and for clearing spaces and energy — a ritual known as 'smudging'. In Shamanic traditions, the sacred wood palo santo is also used as a clearing scent. I don't use it as much now as it is said that the wood has been overused and the demand does not meet the supply. The wood must fall from the tree and be on the ground for four to ten years prior to being harvested. As the demand is higher than the supply, this has resulted in trees being cut down early to meet the demand.

### Himalayan Salt Lamps and Crystals

As mentioned earlier in **Sleep and Circadian Rhythms**, Himalayan salt lamps are great for helping to unwind from the day by bringing a dim, soft, red lighting to the room. They are also known to give off negative ions, a bit like being by the sea, mopping up germs in the air and decreasing allergic irritants. Negative ions help neutralise the positive ions generated from electronics, digital devices and even vacuum cleaners.

*'Negative ions increase the flow of oxygen to the brain, resulting in higher alertness, decreased drowsiness and more mental energy.'* — Pierce J. Howard, PhD, author of *The Owner's Manual for the Brain*

---

37 Professional mendhi artists and incense specialists — www.thehennaden.co.uk

Crystals have great healing properties and benefits but are also very pleasing to the eye and can look stunning as the centrepiece in a home. Here are some of my favourite crystals and their properties:

- Clear quartz — the crystal of higher consciousness; absorbs negative energy
- Amethyst — protector; blocks geopathic stress and negative environmental energies; balances and connects physical, mental and emotional bodies
- Rose quartz — associated with unconditional love; heart opening; infinite peace and self-love (always good to have one in the bedroom)
- Turquoise — spiritual tuning and purification
- Selenite — clarity of mind and higher guidance
- Citrine — powerful cleanser and generator; dissipates negative energy and good for attracting abundance
- Black tourmaline — psychic protection; protects from electro-magnetic smog, cell phones and screens.

When buying crystals, it's better to buy them in person; usually the one you are drawn to is the one for you. Hold it in your hand, close your eyes and see how you feel. If you feel connected and drawn to it, that's the one for you.

### Health Bank Deposits
- ✓ Declutter your space, bag up clothes for charity or sell on eBay — if you haven't worn it in the last 18 months and don't love it, let it go. Go through old photos, keep the ones that hold dear memories. Make a bit of extra money by doing a car boot sale with your stuff. Is there any old paperwork that can be stored as files online?
- ✓ Purify the air in your home by having lots of green plants and foliage
- ✓ Diffuse essential oils and use scents to shift the energy of your home / room
- ✓ Bring Himalayan salt lamps into your home; they act as ionisers and also absorb electromagnetic radiation
- ✓ Crystals make for beautiful decor and have wonderful healing properties

# Electromagnetic Frequencies

Electromagnetic Fields (EMFs) are:

*'Invisible areas of energy, often referred to as radiation that are associated with the use of electrical power.'* — US National Institute of Environmental Health Science

Living in the city, we are surrounded by electromagnetic pollution from power lines, electric circuits in walls, ceilings, floors, electrical appliances, smartphones, computers, Wi-Fi routers, bluetooth headsets, wireless devices, mobile phone masts, smart meters and wireless baby monitors. There is a lot. We are swimming in an invisible sea of EMF.

*'Your body is a complex communication device where cells, tissues, and organs 'talk' to each other to perform basic functions. At each of these levels, the communication includes finely tuned bio-electrical transmitters and receivers, which are almost like tuning into a radio station.'* — Dr Mercola

We are bio-electrical beings; electrical signals are sent out by the heart, lungs and brain to pump blood, breathe and move. Modern technology interferes and disrupts these natural frequencies. In 2011, The World Health Organization (WHO) stated that 'radiofrequency electromagnetic fields as possibly carcinogenic to humans (Group 2B), based on an increased risk for glioma, a malignant type of brain cancer'.[38] People are placing devices close to their body and close to their brain daily, multiple times a day, and even worse, kids are too. Telecommunication companies will still deny mobile phone radiation does any harm to health, just like smoking was deemed safe by tobacco companies in the '50s. The truth is there are thousands of studies in the past decade linking EMFs to negative health effects.

Earlier, I discussed the effects of mobile phone and Wi-Fi radiation on sleep on page 47. In 2016, Dr Martin Pall from Washington State University confirmed that even very low levels of EMF radiation could cause at least 13 mood-disrupting side-effects, including depression,

---

38 International Agency for Research on Cancer: World Health Organization Press Release No 208 (2011) IARC classifies radiofrequency electromagnetic fields as possibly carcinogenic to humans

stress, anxiety and irritability (*Pall, 2016*). Studies published in the *Environment International and Central European Journal of Urology* have also linked low-level electromagnetic radiation from cell phones to an 8% reduction in sperm motility and a 9% reduction in sperm viability. Never carry your cell phone in your pocket (*Adams et al, 2014*). If you do, put it on airplane mode, or make sure you have a protective shield on like Aires Tech®. The same applies to using a laptop or tablet on your lap; keep it away from your body. Those with autoimmune disease or suppressed immune systems may be even more sensitive to EMFs.

Long-term DNA damage caused by radiation from mobile phone and wireless devices was found in the EU REFLEX report in 2004, compiled by 12 scientific institutes from seven different countries.[39] Professor Franz Adlkofer, coordinator of the study stated, 'This is real evidence that hyperfrequency electromagnetic fields can have geno-toxic effects, and this damaged DNA is always the cause of cancer. We've found these damaging effects on the genes at levels well below the safety limits' (*2009*). This research was based on 2G and 3G and now we have much higher levels of radiation with 4G and the forthcoming 5G, which has been deemed a disastrous human experiment on humanity and the environment by scientists.

Living in the city, it's impossible to eliminate exposure to EMFs, but there are ways to greatly reduce your exposure without living off the grid. Follow the health deposits below.

### *Health Bank Deposits*
✓ Turn Wi-Fi off at night and when not in use
✓ Turn off electric sockets in the bedroom at night and, if wires in the walls, turn off sockets in the adjacent room
✓ Video game consoles, Bluetooth dimmer switches, speakers and thermostats and anything wireless emit radio frequency waves 24/7; switch off at night and when not in use
✓ Use an electric/gas oven rather than a microwave
✓ Don't carry your phone on your body or near food or drink; put in a bag or put on airplane mode if in pocket

---

39 Risk evaluation of potential environmental hazards from low energy electromagnetic field (emf) exposure using sensitive in vitro methods — REFLEX REPORT (2004) www.jrseco.com/wp-content/uploads/REFLEX_Final_Report_Part_4.pdf

✓ Use your mobile on speakerphone or a non-wireless headset; avoid holding to the head

✓ Never use a laptop / tablet or smartphone devices on your lap; keep at least one foot away from your body

✓ Reduce time on mobile phone

✓ Get out on your lunch break to a garden, park or patch of grass and put your bare feet on the ground for 30 minutes; the earth is an electrical planet and we are bio-electrical beings. Negative ions from the earth help discharge the positive ions from EMF exposure, helping to harmonise and restore your body's bio-electrical systems

✓ Use a hard-wired baby monitor instead of a wireless one

✓ Avoid smart meters for as long as you can or put a shield on it or shungite rocks next to it (see resources)

✓ When charging devices, keep away from your feet and body, unplug them when not in use as they are a very high source of electric and magnetic fields

✓ Don't charge your mobile phone in your bedroom while you sleep

✓ I have a shield on my devices and wear personal protection from www.airestech.com all independently tested and verified and which I highly recommend. Alternatively, use a Tesla plate for personal protection. You can also get ones to place in your home, car and office (see resources).

✓ Crystals are known EMF absorbers and transmuters. Wear or place them between you and your device and by your Wi-Fi router or put in the corners of your home. Here are some examples:

  ‣ black tourmaline, smoky quartz, black moonstone, amazonite, fluorite, obsidian
  ‣ shungite rock — wear as a pendant and place in corners of your home. It has been said that shungite has protective properties against the harmful effects of electromagnetic radiation, though more research needs to be done
  ‣ orgonites (see resources)

PART 3

# The Soul

# Self Love

As cheesy as it may sound, all relationships start with yourself.

To improve your relationship or attract the relationship you desire you have to deepen the relationship with yourself first. Can you look yourself in the eyes in the mirror and say 'I love you' and mean it? Very few people can. If that feels strange, start with looking at yourself in the mirror every morning; look into your eyes and say: 'I like you and I am open to loving you more'. There is something really special and soul-moving when you take a few quiet moments and space to look yourself in the eyes and say that. It may feel strange and unfamiliar at first but keep doing it to create the habit.

Too often, people look outside themselves to find happiness — in a partner, in consuming and buying 'stuff', in emotional eating and in alcohol and drugs. These are all quick fixes to fill a void. Happiness is a choice and no one is responsible for your happiness. It is not your partner's responsibility to make you happy. It has to come from within'.

You are a complete being, not a half waiting for another half to complete you. You are already complete and when you come together with someone else, the qualities you already have will be amplified. I love watching dating shows, as I spent so many years single and on the dating scene. Often the women interviewed will say: 'I just want to meet someone who makes me happy'. No, be happy first. Be happy with yourself. Find the happiness within and then watch it become amplified when you do meet someone that you are in alignment with.

Self-love is loving *all* of yourself, shadows and all. We all like to present our best foot forward and in the best light. True self-love is loving and embracing all of who we are, the good, the bad and the ugly. That means loving our shadows, the parts of ourselves we suppress and don't want to show to the world — jealousy, judgement, rage, anger, sadness, manipulative behaviour, competitiveness and selfishness. These are all the qualities that would be labelled as 'bad'. Truth is, there is no good or bad, just contrast. If we never felt sadness, we would not know or appreciate the opposite feeling of happiness.

Have you ever noticed that when you try to ignore a feeling, it seems to knock louder and louder on your door? The feeling even creates circumstances, situations, events and people in your life to trigger you to give a voice to it. By choosing to acknowledge and accept your shadow side, it will bring softness to these qualities.

**Exercise**

Identify your top five shadow qualities and reframe them below. Repeat each one out loud as many times as necessary until you feel the emotion soften and feel a sense of acceptance.

*Example:*

▸ 'Even though I am jealous, I love and accept myself anyway'.

Now create your own by filling in the gap with 'I am / I feel' and whatever the shadow emotion you feel most often is.

1. Even though I _____,
   I love and accept myself anyway.

2. Even though I _____,
   I love and accept myself anyway.

3. Even though I _____,
   I love and accept myself anyway.

4. Even though I _____,
   I love and accept myself anyway.

5. Even though I _____,
   I love and accept myself anyway.

A great book to read that goes more into the shadow work is *The Dark Side of the Light Chasers* by Debbie Ford.

**You Are Enough**

You are *enough*, you were born *enough* and everything you need is inside of you. Your power resides within you, not in your job title, salary, marital status or education. Don't let anyone tell you otherwise. When you look at babies and toddlers, they are so joyful, non-judgemental and light up any room. They *know* they are enough, there is never a question or a doubt about that. They are totally present and in the moment. Do you think that as they gurgle away, they are questioning how worthy they are?

It is only through our experiences, social and religious programming and parental conditioning that we may forget the essence of who we truly are — infinite love, here to have a human experience. Our life experiences and failures may knock us down, creating stories that we are not enough. I see failure as life experiences; failures can be our biggest gifts. Most highly successful individuals have failed many times prior to their success like Richard Branson, Walt Disney, JK Rowling, Henry Ford and Thomas Edison, to name but a few. My motto is: 'There is no failure, only feedback'. When Thomas Edison, who invented the electric light bulb, was asked how he felt about failing 10,000 times, his response was: 'I have not failed. I've just found 10,000 ways that won't work'.

Do not see your failures as giving up but as breakthroughs, gifts and life lessons that are steps in your journey to take you to your next adventure. If we can start viewing 'failures' as necessary life lessons we may observe less depression, anxiety and even suicides in school kids and university students under immense pressure to succeed. It's heart-breaking to know that there were 95 suicides of university students in England and Wales between August 2016 to July 2017.[40]

If we can reframe what it means to be successful and reframe failure, instil confidence, self-worth, self-esteem, creativity and a sense of adventure from a young age, I'm certain we will see a dramatic drop in mental health issues for young men and women. I believe it's time for the school system to be revised, prioritising these qualities. We are fortunate to be living in a time where it is possible to do anything you want. It is also the age of the entrepreneur, where it is possible to make a living from what you love. There are kids and

---

40 BBC News; University student suicide rates revealed (2018) - www.bbc.co.uk/news/
   health-44583922

teenagers who are millionaires creating their businesses online, doing what they are passionate about. The age of the traditional working life where you had to go to university and achieve the top grades to get the nine-to-five job with the 'secure' salary that you'd work for the rest of your life is crashing down. Big corporations, the financial and banking system have collapsed. More than ever before, people are working for themselves.

Always remember, *you are enough*. Stick it on a Post-it® note and make it easily visible every day whether on your bathroom mirror, on the wall by your bed and even on your car visor.

*You are enough*

*You were born enough*

*You have always been enough*

You have unique gifts and qualities to bring to the world. Don't spend your whole life trying to fit in, when you were born to stand out.

### Health Bank Deposits
✓ Pick your top five shadow qualities and bring love and acceptance to them
✓ On a Post-it® note, write the affirmation '*I am Enough*' and keep it easily visible

## Play

Too much tension and contraction creates resistance in life. To grow and expand there must be an element of flow. As a perfectionist, over-achiever and striver these qualities are inherent within me and something I've had to learn to become aware of when they start creeping in and creating resistance. Whenever I find myself taking life too seriously, I recognise that I need to add more play and spend time doing something I love that is not related to my business or self-development. I think this is essential for any entrepreneur where your work can be your life. In order to create space for creativity and expansion, it means getting in touch with some right-brain activities such as painting, drawing, games, playing, art, pottery, playing music, working in and dancing.

However, it's important to distinguish that if these activities are taught, they become left-brain activities, so do these activities freely, with no intended goal. The left brain is associated with logic, learning, the rational mind and common sense. Most people are left-brain dominated, with little space for creative ideas, intuition, spontaneous inspiration and receptivity. Play and right-brain activities are vital to induce more flow states and are also the key to manifestation. The 'flow state' or 'being in the zone' is a state of heightened clarity, focus and peak performance. It feels amazing. I feel in a state of flow when I play capoeira, improvising moves in response to the other person's kicks and moves, creating fluidity in movement. It is a true art form. Athletes regularly report being in a flow state during competitions and games.

*'World culture glorifies the hustle and grind, but the grind just isn't sustainable or healthy! The grind is a state of tension and anxiety, feelings of inadequacy and fear. A state in which no amount of effort ever feels enough'.* — Steven Kotler

Flow is the opposite, 'a state of effortless effort', according to Steven Kotler, who committed his life to the scientific study of enhanced states like flow.

Some of my favourite activities that bring an element of play, fun and right-brain activities are:

▸ Capoeira
▸ Dancing
▸ Browsing markets and charity shops
▸ Going to see a musical, dance or circus performance
▸ Bike riding in nature
▸ Watching a comedy
▸ Bringing a sense of play and freestyle movement into physical training
▸ Creating photo collages
▸ Taking time out to meet with like-minded friends where we bounce off each other's energy.

Now it's your turn; list three to five things that bring the element of play and fun into your life. Tuning into having more fun and play opens space for creativity, expansion and growth.

1. _____
2. _____
3. _____
4. _____
5. _____

### Health Bank Deposits

✓ Identify the activities that bring an element of fun and play into your day to activate right-brain thinking
✓ Become aware of when you are taking life too seriously; you'll start feeling tension, contraction and resistance in the flow of life (like you are swimming upstream)
✓ Implement some fun daily

## Your Vibe Attracts Your Tribe

In the animal kingdom, if a mammal is abandoned soon after birth, it stands a low chance of survival. As humans and mammals, we too are hard-wired to connect with others and to be part of a tribe. We all long to form healthy relationships both intimately and socially. Therefore, it's vital to get clear on your own values and priorities (see Part One). Do the people you are spending most of your time with have similar values to you? If you don't know what your values are, you will be attracting random relationships and connections that may not match your pre-defined values because you haven't set them yet.

Those who are with you for what you look like or have will never be by your side forever, but those who are with/around you because they are in alignment with your values, beliefs and common traits will be around much longer. They see you for you, your heart and soul. These are true, deep friendships and relationships, the people who will support you through the good and tough times. Be around those who want to lift you higher, that celebrate your success with you. As you do the inner work on yourself, get aligned with your values and raise your vibe; you may find that people around you drop away because they are no longer in alignment with you. This often happens and is an organic evolution of the path of growth. As the famous quote goes: 'People come into your life for a reason, a season or a lifetime'. This poem by an unknown author sums it up well:

*When you figure out which it is, you know exactly what to do.*

*When someone is in your life for a **reason**, it is usually to meet a need you have expressed outwardly or inwardly. They have come to assist you through a difficulty, to provide you with guidance and support, to aid you physically, emotionally or spiritually. They may seem like a godsend, and they are. They are there for the reason you need them to be. Then, without any wrong doing on your part or at an inconvenient time, this person will say or do something to bring the relationship to an end. Sometimes they die. Sometimes they walk away. Sometimes they act up or out and force you to take a stand. What we must realise is* *that our need has been met, our desire fulfilled; their work is done. The prayer you sent up has been answered and it is now time to move on.*

*When people come into your life for a **season**, it is because your turn has come to share, grow, or learn. They may bring you an experience of peace or make you laugh. They may teach you something you have never done. They usually give you an unbelievable amount of joy. Believe it! It is real! But, only for a season.*

***Lifetime** relationships teach you lifetime lessons; those things you must build upon in order to have a solid emotional foundation. Your job is to accept the lesson, love the person/people (anyway) and put what you have learned to use in all other relationships and areas of your life. It is said that love is blind, but friendship is clairvoyant.* — Author Unknown

Some people come into our lives at different times to help us grow emotionally and spiritually, to share and to learn. This is a good reminder during those challenging times when relationships don't work out or you outgrow your friendship circle. In the past, I went out with a man I had a strong connection with; one minute he thought I was 'the one' and the next, out of the blue, we were done. Weeks later someone else was pregnant with his baby. Although I felt gutted at the time, thank *goodness* that wasn't me and it really reinforced the traits I was looking for in a man. A man with deep integrity, respect and values. This man came into my life for a *reason*. I've had my fair share of Mr Wrongs and heartbreaks. However, each relationship and encounter that didn't work out strengthened my boundaries, got me clearer on my relationship values and ultimately deepened my heart to feel.

The contrast of feeling deep pain expanded my heart to feel deep love. When we reframe our experiences, it softens them, giving space to *feel* the contrasting emotions. When I met my partner Warren, we both had enough life experience to be very clear on what we did and didn't want from a relationship. We had both done the inner work on ourselves separately and were very clear on our values for ourselves and in the relationship we wanted to attract. Through the law of attraction, we found each other and matched what we had both written down about the values of the partner we had wanted to attract! More on the law of attraction later...

### Let Go of People-Pleasing

As hard as it may be to hear, not everyone is going to like you, and that's OK. In my 20s I wanted to be liked by everyone and please everybody, saying yes to everything. People-pleasing is exhausting; do not waste your valuable life force energy doing it because not everyone is going to like you and not everyone is going to agree with your belief systems. You are *enough* and don't need to seek approval or validation from anyone else. Your power is within you, it always has been. Remember your time and energy are the most valuable commodities you have, so choose who you spend your time with and how you spend your time.

While writing this book, I've turned down lots of social events and meeting up with people who want to 'pick my brains' because I had to dedicate time and discipline to writing. Your yes has no power until you say no. Begin to take notice of those who are draining your energy and sucking the life force out of you. You know the ones I mean. We've all been there — where you spend time with certain people and you come back feeling exhausted. This is why it is so important to manage your own energy through breath, meditation, awareness of your thoughts, movement and all the other awesome principles in this book. Some people you must love from a distance and assert boundaries.

### Health Bank Deposits

✓ People come into your life for a reason, season or lifetime — remind yourself of this

✓ Become aware of who you are spending most of your time with; do these relationships feel uplifting or draining? You may have to love some people from a distance or put some boundaries in place

✓ Let go of people-pleasing and saying yes to everyone and everything

# The Art of Letting Go

As human beings we are control freaks. We like to be in control because it keeps us safe. However, it keeps us small too. To live a truly full and expansive life, there has to be an element of surrender to the unknown. As a self-acclaimed perfectionist, that does not come easily to me. When I have let go of pushing, striving and controlling outcomes, I have experienced some of the most magical manifestations of life unfolding. It's one of the hardest things to do, but also the most liberating, and it's an ongoing work in progress for me. Transformational Breath® has been a game-changer for me, allowing me to ultimately open more to life.

*'Letting go is hard but sometimes holding on is harder.'*

Nothing is certain in life. We will lose people we love, people will die, we may have our hearts broken, jobs may not last forever, we will get hurt, relationships may break down. There is one thing for certain for all of us — we will pass on from our physical bodies. Be in the *now*; celebrate life, stop holding on to the past, let go of certainty and embrace the magic of life that awaits you.

I've worked with clients who are stuck in jobs they hated but stayed for the security, the fear of the unknown being too much for them. Yet they could be made redundant or have their job cut any time in the future. Look what happened to the entire financial system in 2007. Nothing is guaranteed. Life is constantly moving and unfolding and so are you. Let go, surrender and allow yourself to bring more flow and magic into your life. To truly let go is to become detached from the outcome.

*'Let go of what was, accept what is and surrender to what will be...'*

Depression is living in the past and anxiety fearing the future. As neuroscientist Dr Joe Dispenza beautifully puts it, you create your future from the unpredictable, i.e., the unknown.

I highly recommend *The Surrender Experiment* by Michael A Singer. It's a true story of how the author's life becomes an experiment of surrender. He manifests the most incredible, divinely orchestrated opportunities, relationships and meetings, including building a billion-dollar software company from scratch, having had no experience in software!

> *'At some point there is no more struggle, just a deep peace that comes from surrendering to a perfection that is beyond your comprehension. Eventually, even the mind stops resisting. The joy, excitement and freedom are simply too beautiful to give up. Once you are ready to let go of yourself, life becomes your friend, your teacher, your secret lover. When life's way becomes your way, all the noise stops, and there is a great peace.'* —
> Michael A. Singer

### Forgiveness

Holding on to past hurts and resentment creates disharmony in the body and mind, keeping you stuck. It is said 'withholding forgiveness is like drinking poison and waiting for the other person to die' (author unknown). Forgiveness does not mean condoning or dismissing another's behaviour but instead freedom from carrying the burdens of the past, creating more space to move forward in life. It is easy to get caught up in the stories, patterns and the associated familiar emotions, but remember you create your future from the unknown space unfolding in front of you. When we let go, we make space to create. Forgiveness can take time but, ultimately, will lead you to feeling freer and lighter. Try this forgiveness meditation and repeat as often as necessary.

### Forgiveness Meditation

*Imagine yourself standing at the top of a beautiful mountain, the sun is shining down on you and brings warmth to your face. The sky is clear and blue; you take a deep breath inhaling the fresh, mountainous, clear air that nourishes you from within. As you look behind you, you see people from your life experience and from the past walking up the mountain to greet you. They begin to line up in front of you. Your spouse, partner, ex-spouse, ex-partner, mother, father, siblings, children, other family members, teachers, boss, ex-boss, ex-lover, business partners and colleagues. They have come to receive your forgiveness.*

*As you stand in your power on top of the mountain, see the first person coming up, see them standing in their own power, look this person in the eyes and say, 'I forgive you and release you'. You have nothing but warm thoughts and good intentions for this person as you see them in a bubble of light float away from you and continue on their journey. Breathing deeply, continue onto each person as they come forward, repeating 'I forgive you and release you'. As they stand before you, if there feels like a powerful energetic charge, visualise a cord connecting your heart to theirs. As you repeat to yourself 'I forgive you and release you', visualise the cord being cut by a sword from your end and their end, disconnecting you from their energy immediately and releasing them. Send them back down the mountain. Continue this as many times as you like until you feel a sense of lightness. Some may need to get in line more than once!*

*When you have finished with everyone in line, look to see a small person walking up the mountain towards you. It is YOU, as a child. Have that child stand before you and look directly into his/her eyes and say: 'I love you and forgive you for I have looked into your heart and I see you are innocent'. Give that child whatever it needs at this time, whatever messages he/she needs to hear. Then wrap that child in your arms and hold them repeating: 'I love you and forgive you for I have looked into your heart and see you are innocent'. When you are complete, bring your awareness back to your environment and make any notes in your journal.*

### Health Bank Deposits

- ✓ Adopt the mantra 'I let go of what was, I accept what is, I surrender to what will be'
- ✓ Do the forgiveness meditation as many times as you need
- ✓ Read *The Surrender Experiment* by Michael A Singer

## The Law of Attraction

*'Like attracts like.'*

Quantum physics says that everything is energy, that everything in the universe is made up of vibrating particles and energy vibrating at different frequencies, including you. Everything is constantly moving and vibrating at one speed or another. The entire universe is made up of atoms, including *you*, and science has shown that these atoms are continually vibrating and oscillating. All solid, liquid and gas is made up of atoms vibrating at different speeds. Think about how radio waves are transmitted to your radio — they come through waves of frequencies travelling through solid and matter that we cannot see but enable you to tune in.

I first came across the law of attraction through the book *The Secret*, which is a great introduction to the philosophy; however it does not emphasise the importance of feelings. Your thoughts and feelings create your reality; where your attention goes, energy flows. Your brain is a powerful transmitter; its electromagnetic field frequency conducts through solid and matter. Within you, you have your very own GPS system (your emotional guidance system) navigating you in life. Your thoughts, emotions and how you feel determine what you attract into your life. There is always a choice; you can change how you think and feel and rewire the brain for new experiences, thought patterns and belief systems. We've already discussed the power of your thoughts in Part One and the impact it has on emotional health and biochemistry.

We are electrical, vibrational beings and the frequency you are vibrating at will attract the people, circumstances, events and situations vibrating at that same frequency. To really attract what you want in your life you must take responsibility to raise your vibration and get aligned so that you can manifest the reality you desire. The key here is *responsibility*; blaming others for your misfortunes or things not working out as you would like keeps you in a victim consciousness vibrating at a low level. Instead, what are the lessons you can take from your misfortunes or failures, even the really challenging times in your life? As Tony Robbins says: 'Life is happening *for* you, not *to* you'.

### How The Law of Attraction Works

What you *think* and *feel* most of the time creates your reality. If you are constantly having disempowering self-talk, feel grumpy and angry at the world and believe that good things never happen for you, you are literally training your brain and heart to believe this is true, emitting powerful signals into the world transmitting from your brain and heart into your energy field. Research by HeartMath® has found the pattern of your heart rhythm reflects the state of your emotions and nervous system dynamics.[41] Your heart sends coherent signals to the brain when feeling positive emotions such as appreciation, joy, love, happiness and the brain synchronises to the heart's coherent rhythm.

The brain does not know the difference between what is real and what isn't. When emitting these signals into the world, it must manifest back to match the frequency being emitted. In this example situations, circumstances, experiences, people and events may show up in life that evoke more anger against the world, apparently validating the belief of some people that good things never happen for them. This is why we see people repeating the same patterns, relationships, circumstances etc., until they break the loop, change the thought, how they feel and break old belief systems. Simply start by getting into the feeling of feeling good; feel good within yourself. There are plenty of practices in this book to help you do that. By managing your energy first, you are raising your frequency.

Ever notice how some people seem to have all the luck? There is no such thing as luck; you create your reality. These people who seem to have it all, usually have a very positive, clear mindset; they feel good about themselves and there seems to be something about them that is infectious and draws people to them.

---

41 The Science of heart math (2019) - www.heartmath.com/science/

Dr Masaru Emoto, New York best-selling author of *The Hidden Messages in Water,* conducted ground-breaking research into the vibration of words, thoughts, intentions, sound and its effect on water (*Emoto, 2004*). He observed through microscopic photography beautiful geometric crystallisations that would form in the water when positive words such as 'thank you', 'love' and 'peace' were written on a label and put around the bottles of water. Negative words had the opposite effect, distorting the crystal-like structures in the water. In essence, words, thoughts and intentions carry a vibration that affects the molecular structure of water. As humans are made up of 70% water, it is crucial to be constantly aware of the words spoken, and thoughts and intentions you have.

### Emotional Guidance Scale

I also believe you can't fake how you feel. If you feel you can't move to a place of feeling good just yet by doing the things that bring you joy, then look at raising your frequency to the next emotion on the emotional guidance scale opposite (created by Esther and Jerry Hicks). For example, if you are feeling disappointment, can you transcend and move it to frustration / irritation by focusing on another thought that relieves the feeling of disappointment? This way, you are on your way to moving up the emotional guidance scale and getting into alignment with your heart's desires.

**High Vibration 1 – 7**

High emotion = strong attraction, getting what you want (the better it gets, the better it gets)

1. Joy / Appreciation / Empowered / Freedom / Love
2. Passion
3. Enthusiasm / Eagerness / Happiness
4. Positive Expectation / Belief
5. Optimism
6. Hopefulness
7. Contentment
8. Boredom
9. Pessimism
10. Frustration / Irritation / Impatience
11. Overwhelment
12. Disappointment
13. Doubt
14. Worry
15. Blame
16. Discouragement
17. Anger
18. Revenge
19. Hatred / Rage
20. Jealousy
21. Insecurity / Guilt / Unworthiness
22. Fear / Grief / Depression / Despair / Powerlessness

**Low Vibration 8 – 22**

High emotion = strong attraction; getting what you don't want (the worse it gets, the worse it gets)

\* Taken from *Ask and It Is Given* by Esther and Jerry Hicks

Are you ready to create your reality? What do you wish to attract in your life? Is it love? A romantic partner? More clients? Business opportunities? Deeper connecting friendships?

1. What do you want to attract into your life? Focus on one thing.
   *For example, more clients and business opportunities that are aligned with your vision.*

   _____

   _____

   _____

2. Can you tap into the emotion of how it would make you feel?
   *For example, excited and joyful.*

   _____

   _____

   _____

3. Get into the practice of raising your vibration. What makes you feel good?
   *For example, I love to put some music on and dance.*
   List three things that can be your go-to, instantly raising your vibration.

   _____

   _____

   _____

### Health Bank Deposits

- ✓ Identify one thing you want to attract into your life and how it would make you feel
- ✓ List three things that make you feel good as they raise your vibration
- ✓ Practice an attitude of gratitude (Part One). Appreciation is number one on the Emotional Guidance Scale.

# Vision and Dream Building

Now that you understand the power of your thoughts and the law of attraction, it's time to create your reality and manifest your dreams through creating a vision / dream board. A vision / dream board is a collage of images, quotes and affirmations that focus on your dreams and desires, serving as inspiration and using the law of attraction to bring your vision to fruition. I am a big fan of vision boards. My group of close friends and I have been doing vision boards for the past ten years. I have found them to be very powerful and have manifested incredible opportunities. For years I dreamt of splitting my life between London and working abroad on retreats in beautiful locations. I manifested working on retreats and events in Turkey, Portugal, Morocco, Norway and Italy. While working on a retreat in Portugal, when I stood on the yoga deck, I had a feeling of deja vu. It was in fact a mirror image of a picture I had put on my board a few years earlier that I found on the internet.

Prior to that, I had been turned down from other retreats and opportunities but, as I got clearer on the lifestyle I wanted to achieve, I put images of being outdoors in nature, beautiful locations, delicious healthy foods and juices and doing yoga in nature. The more I saw these images, the closer it felt to my reality until it had to manifest. It's important to remember as you look at the images on your board that you feel good. Let the positive emotions and feelings of gratitude you evoke from looking at the images fill you up. When you feel the emotions, the brain does not know the difference between what's real and what's not, and soon the reality will be attracted into your life like a magnet to match the vibration you are emitting.

A friend, Guy, encouraged me to add something that I'd like to do, but perhaps could not easily go out and do. I put husky sledding, as it's something I'd love to do but not something I would plan to, as when I travel, I like to go to hot places. A few years later, however, I manifested an incredible opportunity to go to the Arctic for a few days for a fitness and yoga well-being trip. The yoga teacher had to drop out at the last minute and I was asked 24 hours before if I could go out and teach. It was an opportunity of a lifetime so of course I said *yes*. One of the activities on offer was husky sledding in the Arctic Circle. It was magical; the location was totally unspoilt, and it felt like I was in Narnia. I had manifested beyond what I could ever have imagined. This is what happens time and time again when you let go of any perceived outcome.

### Creating Your Dream / Vision Board
You will need
- Scissors
- Glue / drawing pins
- Pictures that inspire you — from magazines or the internet
- A3-size, or bigger, thick card / cork noticeboard

Your main vision board focuses on all areas of your life. Think about the goals in your life for your career, relationships, finances, home, travel, health, spirituality and social life. Focus on how you want to feel and what inspires you. I have photos of fond memories with friends and handwritten affirmations such as, 'I am healthy, radiant and vibrant'. I have inspirational quotes from people I admire like Marianne Williamson, and some handwritten financial and career goals. Some questions you may want to ask yourself to help you create your vision board are:

- *What do you wish to bring into your life?*
- *How do you want to feel?*
- *What makes you feel good?*
- *What do you desire?*
- *What / who inspires you?*

If there is one area of your life you feel needs particular focus and more energy directed to it, create a smaller theme board. For example, when I was looking for a property to buy within a certain budget, I created a board focused on the home I wanted to attract, the price range, accessibility, certain features etc. Once I let go of the fear of investing all my money, I attracted the home that ticked all the boxes.

I recommend creating your board by hand rather than a digital board; this helps you to get into the process of creating as using your hands to cut and stick images brings it to life more. Have it in a space you can see it readily, because what you focus on expands, helping to bring the visions into your reality. Remember the art of letting go — letting go of how it will manifest but sitting in how good it makes you *feel*.

Set aside an hour or two, put some music on and get creating. Even invite some friends over and get co-creating; doing it in a group amplifies the intentions and visions you set. Your dreams may change over time and new inspirations will come in, so update whenever you feel the need to. I'd love to know how you get on; post your vision board and tag me @wholisticbodylife on Instagram. Putting your vision out to the world is a powerful declaration to the universe.

### Health Bank Deposits

✓ Create your vision board

✓ Place it somewhere you can readily see it

✓ Tag me on Instagram / Facebook with a picture of your vision board @wholisticbodylife

## Putting It All Together

For some of you, reading this book will serve as a gentle reminder to get back on track, and for others it may be a complete lifestyle overhaul. Take your time working through this book. I suggest implementing the easiest and simplest changes first, the ones that you will and can do. It's already overwhelming enough living in the city, so implement the things that are most doable first until they become ingrained as a habit. For example, everyone can switch their Wi-Fi off before bed and turn their mobile phone on airplane mode.

Go through the exercises in the book and refer to the Health Bank Deposits at the end of each section. It's about having more deposits than withdrawals in your health bank account. As you start to top up your account and make the necessary changes, you will be much better off physically, emotionally, mentally and spiritually. Don't try to do everything all at once and create a more overwhelming situation. You'll feel what resonates most with you, so let your inner wisdom guide you to the changes and actions you need to prioritise.

## Creating a Morning/Evening Ritual

You may have heard that most successful entrepreneurs and business leaders have a morning routine/ritual. Hal Elrod, best-selling author of *The Miracle Morning*, says how you start your day largely determines the quality of your day, your work and your life (*Elrod, 2016*). How you start your day is *key* to how the rest of your day unfolds. Starting your day from a grounded and centred place is essential to mental and spiritual health. Imagine how your relationship to everything changes when you are serving from a more grounded place — the relationship to yourself, your partner, children, clients and colleagues. Having a morning routine helps you to be more present, less reactive and more responsive. Starting your day by managing your own energy first is transformational and should be a priority, especially if you are a coach, health practitioner, teacher or in the profession of helping others. You must fill yourself up first so that you can be in a place to serve. So many people wake up to checking their phone, emails and notifications. Straight away they are putting themselves in a reactive state and at the service of others, before they've given any time for themselves. Don't check your phone until you have completed your morning routine.

Begin by choosing *one* thing to focus on in the morning. It could be meditation, diaphragmatic breathing, affirmations, gratitude journaling or the work in programme. Start with five minutes and get disciplined in doing this daily until it becomes a habit. If you miss a day, don't worry. Don't beat yourself up but get back on track the next day. The benefits are cumulative so just be consistent.

Managing my energy and emotional state first thing in the morning is so ingrained that it is now non-negotiable for me. There is not much that will get in the way of that. In time, work up to building a 20-minute morning routine into your daily life. Mine consists of five minutes of breathwork/gratitude journaling followed by 15–20 minutes of meditation. I have many tools to pick from now that I intuitively choose what I feel I need most each morning, so I rotate the tools I have. Sometimes it's mobility movement followed by meditation. Some mornings I can spend up to an hour on my morning ritual incorporating movement, breathwork, meditation, affirmations and gratitude. Set yourself a challenge of 30 days to get started and tag me with your morning ritual @wholisticbodylife on Instagram. I'd love to hear about it.

For the evening, follow my wind-down routine in Part Two — **Sleep and Circadian Rhythms** to help facilitate deep, restful sleep. It's important to have some time to switch off from the day too without relying on a glass of wine or beer each evening as that can soon turn into a bad habit. I always say to my clients, if you go to bed in a bad mood, you wake up in a bad mood. Take some time to wind down and change your state. Just ten slow diaphragmatic breaths have been shown to relax the entire nervous system and lower blood pressure.

## End Note

As humans we are here on earth to have an experience. You are here now in this lifetime; this lifetime will not last forever. Enjoy the now, enjoy the moment, be present. Do the things that make your heart sing, dance like nobody's watching, love deeply and passionately, spend time with those who lift you up and inspire you, feel the power of your spirit in your breath, feel a breeze brush against your face and the sun touching your skin. Tune into the miracle it is to be a human being. As one of my coaches says, 'You will f*** up, make mistakes and get things wrong and that's OK'. You are human so learn from them. Life is not a dress rehearsal, this is the real thing and there is no manual!

From surviving to thriving, may this book inspire you to live a healthy, happy and full life in alignment with your values and dreams.

In health and happiness,

Francesca xxx

# Acknowledgements

First and foremost, my partner Warren — thank you for letting me interrupt you with whatever you were doing at any given time and listen to me read out loud passages during the writing process! Thank you for your love, patience and continuous support in my growth. You inspire me daily with your life's work as a dedicated holistic lifestyle and spiritual coach who truly embodies and lives the values you teach.

My amazing sister and number one fan, Danni Blechner and the team at Conscious Dreams Publishing — thank you! Danni, you were the person who pushed me to write a book and to self-publish through you is truly very special. I know how proud you are of me, 'your little sister', and I am so happy to have the support of you and your team through the publishing process.

Thank you, Paul Chek, for your teachings on which much of this book is based. Your teachings of holistic health and the importance of mental, emotional, spiritual and physical health has profoundly shaped the way I work with my clients. To Jo Rushton, my teacher on Holistic Lifestyle Coaching Level 2, for using me as a case study — another pivotal moment in my life that forced me to re-evaluate the pace I was living at, how ungrounded I was and how close I was to burnout. To Douglas Heel — thank you for your profound teachings of Be Activated Techniques that first highlighted to me how 'scattered' my physiology and nervous system was.

Nathalie Montille, my incredible Transformational Breath® trainer — you emit such unconditional love and power and you helped lead me to shine my light and stand in my power. Thank you for your role in my life at a time of immense growth, healing and transformation. To Elif Clarke, my Transformational Breath® mentor — thank you for your laughs, jokes, support and for always championing me along (and driving off without me — couldn't resist!). To Rebecca Dennis — thank you for your friendship, love, support and inspiration with your breath work, for trusting me to work so closely with you and passing opportunities my way when I was starting out. To my incredible female spiritual warrior coaches and mentors, Jody Shield and Alexi Panos — you have inspired me greatly as a female entrepreneur to live in alignment with my values and dreams and shown me that anything is possible. Love you guys.

To Maiya Leeke — thank you for sharing your story and for our connection ever since the retreat in Portugal. Your challenges, your approach and resilience in life inspire both Warren and I. You have created your own youth dance company and passed on the teachings of mindset, positive affirmations and the breath and are empowering young people through dance even when you were facing such challenges yourself. You are such an inspiration to us through all you have endured; you are going to change the world. We love you.

To my Mum — thank you for always championing me and for introducing us to alternative and complementary health when we were younger. Thank you for your strength, wisdom and robust genes and for encouraging me to follow my passion and do what I love. To my Dad — thank you for your kindness. Finally, to my grandmother who is my spirit guide — a powerful, strong woman whose presence lives through me, guiding me in my life to do what I love.

To my ancestors that have passed after enduring real hardships — you have carved the path for me to live my life, create my legacy and make a difference in people's lives. I honour you.

## About the Author

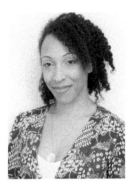

Francesca lives in London and is the founder of Wholistic Body Life which provides a holistic and integrative health approach to restoring harmony and balance in a fast-paced world.

Having been on the edge of burnout many times in the past as a personal trainer, she became passionate about helping others self-restore and thrive physically, mentally, emotionally and spiritually. Using her 20 years' worth of experience in fitness, holistic health and well-being, she founded her company to help others live healthier, happier and more fulfilled lives.

Along the way, she has helped thousands of people from all over the world and all walks of life. These include members of the Saudi Royal Family, celebrities, business leaders, new mothers and teenagers. She works with her clients one-on-one or in group settings either face-to-face or virtually, runs group workshops and events and works on local and international retreats.

Francesca has also featured in the local London news and on national radio. Her loves are dark chocolate, trawling vintage markets and travelling.

www.wholisticbodylife.com

wholisticbodylife

wholistic body life

# Resources

1. www.abelandcole.co.uk enter 738366 for your first FREE box
2. www.bambooclothing.co.uk — enter Francesca Blechner at CHECKOUT for 15% off first order
3. www.beejameditation.com
4. www.breastcancer.org.uk/reduce-your-risk/are-you-being-exposed/
5. www.breastcanceruk.org.uk/reduce-your-risk/chemicals-and-environment/
6. www.breastcanceruk.org.uk/app/uploads/2019/09/A-to-Z-Chemicals-of-ConcernWeb.pdf
7. www.breastcanceruk.org.uk/app/uploads/2019/08/BCUK_EDC_brief_v2_20.9.1pdf
8. www.chekinstitute.com
9. C.H.E.K Institute Advanced Training Programs- Holistic Lifestyle Coaching www.chekinstitute.com/chek-holistic-lifestyle-coach-program/
10. Find a CHEK Practitioner near you www.chekconnect.com/app/findpractitioner
11. C.H.E.K Institute
    3145 Tiger Run Court, Suite 101
    Carsbad, CA 92010
    U.S.A.
    CHEK Europe Ltd.
    2 Lawrence Lane
    Eccleston
    Chorley, Lancashire
    PR7 5SJ
12. www.drmercola.com
13. www.ewg.org/foodnews/clean-fifteen.php
14. www.ewg.org/foodnews/dirty-dozen.php
15. www.ewg.org/skin deep/top-tips-for-safer-products/

16. www.farmdrop.com
17. www.findaspring.com
18. www.thehennaden.co.uk
19. www.holisticsonline.com/earthing-and-emf/tesla — enter my practitioner code PRACT30
20. www.holisticsonline.com/earthing-and-emf/orgone — enter my practitioner code PRACT30
21. www.litethelight.bigcartel.com/intention
22. www.lfm.org.uk/
23. www.themindfulchef.com
24. www.mydoterra.com/wholisticbodylife/#/
25. www.nealsyardremedies.com
26. www.riverford.co.uk
27. www.rootandflower.co.uk
28. www.secretldn.com/stunning-green-spaces-london/
29. www.soilassociation.org
30. www.theorganicpharmacy.com/expert-tips/carcinogens
31. www.transformationalbreath.com
32. www.veggiwash.co.uk/
33. www.youtube.com/watch?v=MOLike-Hkpg

# References

Abou-Donia MB, El-Mastry EM, Abdel-Rahman AA, et al (2008) Splenda alters gut microflora and increases intestinal p-glycoprotein and cytochrome p-450 in male rats. *Journal of Toxicology and Environmental Health 71:21; 1415 – 29*

Adams JA, Galloway TS, Mondal D, et al (2014) Effect of mobile telephones on sperm quality: a systematic review and meta-analysis. *Journal of Environment International 70; 106 – 112*

Adlkofer, F (2009) How susceptible are genes to mobile phone radiation? *www.jrseco.com/wp-content/uploads/how-susceptible-are-genes-to-mobile-phone-radiation-adlkofer-kompetenz.pdf*

Barański M, Średnicka-Tober D, Volakakis N, et al (2014) Higher antioxidant and lower cadmium concentrations and lower incidence of pesticide residues in organically grown crops: a systematic literature review and meta-analyses. *British Journal of Nutrition 112:5; 794 – 811*

Barry V, Winquist A, Steenland K (2013) Perfluorooctanoic acid (PFOA) exposures and incident cancers among adults living near a chemical plant. *Journal of Environmental Health Perspectives 121:11 – 12; 1313 – 1318*

Byrne, R (2006) *The Secret.* Beyond Words, New York

Capaldo A, Gay F, Lepretti M, Paolella G, et al (2018) Effects of environmental cocaine concentrations on the skeletal muscle of the European eel (Anguilla Anguilla). *Journal of Science of the Total Environment 1; 640 – 1*

Chek, P (2004) *How to Eat, Move and Be Healthy.* C.H.E.K Institute, San Diego, CA

Chek, P (2012) Breathing and Movement. www.paulcheksblog.com/breathing-and-movement-2/

DeBakey M, et al (1964) *Journal of American Medical Association 189; 655 – 59*

Defarge N, Spiroux de Vendômois J, Séralini GE (2018) Toxicity of formulants and heavy metals in glyphosate-based herbicides and other pesticides. *Journal of Toxicology Reports 5; 156 – 163*

Dyer, W (2012) *Two Little Words! The Power of I Am.* www.healyourlife.com/two-little-words

Elrod, H (2016) *The Miracle Morning,* Hodder and Stoughton, London

Emoto, M (2004) *The Hidden Messages in Water.* Beyond Words, New York

Fong Ha, S (1996) *Yiquan and The Nature of Energy — the fine art of doing nothing and achieving everything.* Summerhouse Publications, Berkeley, CA

Freud, S (2001) *The Standard Edition of the Complete Psychological Works of Sigmund Freud. On the History of the Post Psychoanalytic Movement, papers on Metapsychology and other works (1914 – 1916).* Hogarth Press, London

Getoff, David (2001) *Attaining Optimal Health in the 21st Century.* Videocassette series.

Golomb, BA (1998) Cholesterol and Violence: Is there a connection? *Annals of Internal Medicine Journal 28:6; 478 – 87*

Hamilton, D (2017) *The Five Side Effects of Kindness.* Hay House, London

Hicks, J & E (2009) *Ask and it is Given, Learning to Manifest the Law of Attraction.* Hayhouse, London

Hoekzema E, Barba-Müller E, Pozzobon C, et al (2017) Pregnancy leads to long lasting changes in human brain structure. *Nature Neuroscience Journal 20; 287 – 296*

Hoffman, B The Influence of Sugar and Artificial Sweeteners on Vascular Health during the Onset and Progression of Diabetes. *www.plan.core-apps.com/eb2018/abstract/382e0c7eb95d6e76976fbc663612d58a*

Hölzel BK, et al (2011) Mindfulness practice leads to increases in regional brain grey matter density. *Journal of Psychiatry Research: Neuroimaging, 191:1; 36 – 43*

Howard, PJ (2006) *The Owner's Manual for the Brain: Everyday applications from mind brain research.* Bard Press, Austin, TX

Jewell, T (2018) *'What is Diaphragmatic Breathing'* www.healthline.com/health/diaphragmatic-breathing

Keys A, Aravanis C, Blackburn HW, et al (1966) Epidemiological studies related to coronary heart disease. Characteristics of men aged 40–59 in Seven Countries. *Acta Medica Scandinavica 460:1–392*

Knutson KL and Cauter EV (2015) Associations between sleep loss and increased risk of obesity and diabetes www.ncbi.nlm.nih.gov/pmc/articles/PMC4394987/

Kotler, S (2019) How Peak Performance expert Steven Kotler enters the Flow State https://blog.mindvalley.com/flow-state/

Krüger M, Schledorn P, Schrödl W, et al (2014) Detection of Glyphosate Residues in Animals and Humans. *Journal of Environmental and Analytical Toxicology, 4; 210*

Lazar SW, Kerr CE, Wasserman RH, et al (2005) Meditation Experience is associated with increased cortical thickness. *Neuroreport 16:17; 1893–1897*

Mazurek, A How to Breathe Better to Move Better. www.chekinstitute.com/blog/how-to-breathe-better-to-move-better/

Mercola, J (2010) The Cholesterol Myth That is Harming your Health. articles.mercola.com/sites/articles/archive/2010/08/10/making-sense-of-your-cholesterol-numbers.aspx

Mercola, J (2011) Saturated Fat: The Forbidden Food you should never stop eating articles.mercola.com/sites/articles/archive/2011/09/01/enjoy-saturated-fats-theyre-good-for-you.aspx

(Dr) Mercola's Six Key Principles *https://shop.mercola.com/pages/dr-mercolas-six-key-principles*

Mercola, J (2016) An Inside Look into the Fish Industry Reveals Disturbing Facts That Could Threaten Your Health. *https://articles.mercola.com/sites/articles/archive/2016/04/30/salmon-fish-farming.aspx*

Mesnage R, Defarge N, Spiroux de Vendômois J, et al (2014) Major Pesticides Are More Toxic to Human Cells Than Their Declared Active Principles. *BioMed Research International, Article ID 179691*

Ohayon, MM and Milesi, C (2016) Artificial Outdoor Nighttime Lights Associate with Altered Sleep Behavior in the American General Population. *Journal of Sleep 39:6; 1311 – 1320*

Pall, ML (2016) Microwave frequency electromagnetic fields (EMFs) produce widespread neuropsychiatric effects including depression. *Journal of Chemical Neuroanatomy 75; 43 – 51*

Portas CM, Bjorvatn B, Ursin R (2000) Serotonin and the sleep/wake cycle: special emphasis on microdialysis studies. *Journal of Progress in Neurobiology, 60; 13 – 35*

Ravnskov, U (1998) The questionable role of saturated and polyunsaturated fatty acids in cardiovascular disease. *Journal of Clinical Epidemiology 51; 443 – 60*

Reichelt KL, Lindback T, Scott H, (1994) Increased levels of antibodies to food proteins in Down syndrome. *Japanese Pediatric Journal 36; 489 – 492*

Schmid, SM, Hallschmid M, Jauch-Chara K, et al (2008) A Single night of sleep deprivation increases ghrelin levels and feelings of hunger in normal healthy weight men. *Journal of Sleep Research 3; 331 – 4*

Shattock P, Kennedy A, Rowell F, et al (1990) Role of neuropeptides in autism and their relationship with classical neurotransmitters. *Brain Dysfunction 3:5; 328 – 45*

Shuster KA, Brock KL, Dysko RC et al (2012) Polytetrafluoroethylene Toxicosis in Recently Hatched Chickens (Gallus domesticus). *Journal of Comparative Medicine 62:1; 49 – 52*

Simopoulos, AP (2016) An increase in the Omega-6/Omega-3 Fatty acid ratio increases the risk for obesity. *Nutrients 8:3; 128*

Singer, MA (2015) *The Surrender Experiment*. Yellow Kite, UK

Średnicka-Tober D, Marcin M, Seal CJ, et al (2016) Composition differences between organic and conventional meat: a systematic literature review and meta-analysis. *British Journal of Nutrition 115:6; 994 – 1011*

Średnicka-Tober D, Marcin M, Seal CJ, et al (2016) Higher PUFA and n-3 PUFA, conjugated linoleic acid, α-tocopherol and iron, but lower iodine and selenium concentrations in organic milk: a systematic literature review and meta- and redundancy analyses. *British Journal of Nutrition 115:6; 1043 – 1060*

Steegmans PH, Hoes AW, Bak AA, et al (2000) Higher prevalence of depressive symptoms in middle-aged men with low serum cholesterol levels. *Journal of Psychosomatic Medicine 62:2; 205 – 11*

Strauss, R (2016) *Natural Household Cleaning.* IMM Lifestyle Books, UK

Tracy, B (2003) *Change your Thinking, Change your Life.* John Wiley & Sons, Hoboken, NJ

Van Der Kolk, B (2015) *The Body Keeps the Score.* Penguin Random House, USA.

Wood B, Rea M, Plitnick B, Figueiro M, (2012) Light level and duration of exposure determine the impact of self-luminous tablets on melatonin suppression. *Journal of Applied Ergonomics 44:2; 237 – 240*

Zaltman, G (2003) *How Customers Think: Essential Insights into the Mind of the Market.* Harvard Business School Publishing, Boston, MA

# Recommended Reading

Bradley P, Journey CA, Button DT, et al (2016) Metformin and other Pharmaceuticals widespread in wadeable streams of the Southeastern United States. *Environmental Science and Technology Letters 3:6; 243 – 249*

Ford, D (2001) *The Dark Side of the Light Chasers.* Hodder and Stoughton, London

Hall, J (2009) *The Crystal Bible.* Godsfield Press, London

Hill, N (2007) *Think and Grow Rich.* First edition, Wilder Publications, Virginia

Kendrick, M (2007) *The Great Cholesterol Con.* John Blake Publishing, UK

Munro K, Martins C, Loewenthal M, et al (2019) Evaluation of combined sewer overflow impacts on short-term pharmaceutical and illicit drug occurrence in a heavily urbanised tidal river catchment (London, UK). *Science of The Total Environment 657; 1099 – 111*

Pineault, N (2017) The Non-Tinfoil Guide to EMF's. N & G Media www.nontinfoilemf.com

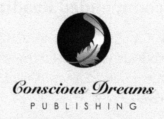

## Conscious Dreams
### PUBLISHING

*Be the author of your own destiny*

Find out about our authors, events, services
and how you too can get your book journey started.

f  Conscious Dreams Publishing

𝕏  @DreamsConscious

📷  @consciousdreamspublishing

in  Daniella Blechner

www  www.consciousdreamspublishing.com

✉  info@consciousdreamspublishing.com

*Let's connect*

Connection

* proactive about connecting w/ ppl who interest me

* allow space/distance from old/tired connections — allow room for New

* 80/20 rule — it's ok to connect with 20% who are not on totally right wavelength for me — because I recognise value in good ppl, with good hearts, who stand the test of time. I don't get fixated on all ppl being on the right wavelength

* weekly I connect with the 80%
  - a day in London/outside of Luton
  - a friend/client/colleague
    eg TrBT
  - dates/fun activities
    w/ Ben.
  - a therapist/facilitator → it still counts!!

~

Wellness

* I strip back to do list & expectations of myself. I don't create hectioness in my week, in my day. I create steady progress + room.

* I charge for my time. I tell clients this will take longer. I track my _time_ & charge for most of it. 80/20 rule. I only don't charge when it secures future work... I charge for meetings post 'kick-off.

* I do not fear new projects because I tackle them ALL in line with my daily schedule
  - work time    - creative time
  - email time
  - me time.

& because I update clients & be transparent around time/costs — I will always be respected & renumerated this way.

* I keep some days 100% ~~free~~

* I ~~forward~~ plan massage, breath appointments, walks in nature. I 'routine-ize' this stuff!!!

* I ~~forward~~ plan a walk daily. This is a big charge. But will make the most difference.

It can be some other kind of
"in nature" pursuit eg open water
swim.

* I keep studying, learning.

Creativity * Throw It Down is a key project

* I routinize creativity by adding it
/scheduling it

* I more mindfully choose my
projects, to include exciting,
'stretch' projects eg writing
my own book, stories, making
our poetry, music, saving for a
2nd home I can create/decorate
wildly!!

* Incidental creativity + Intentional
creativity.

* I sort out my artist channel
online to receive my highest
good

* I blend music & breath